Praise for
Kinship Medicine

"If there's a word for the sickness that plagues our country, it's hyper-individualism—and happily, as this fine book makes clear, there's a cure: Connection. Relationship. Communion. Read this book—optimally in the company of others!"

 —BILL MCKIBBEN, author of *The Flag, the Cross, and the Station Wagon*

"In an age of disconnection, Wendy Johnson offers a vital prescription for both personal and planetary flourishing. By bridging ancient wisdom and modern science, she offers a fresh and deeply human perspective on thriving in today's world. *Kinship Medicine* is the kind of book that stays with you long after you've turned the final page."

 —DANIEL H. PINK, #1 *New York Times* best-selling author of *Drive* and
  The Power of Regret

"Such an important book for our time, for all times. We have much to discover about our body and the body of this earth and the profound connection between the two. This book opens those interconnected worlds for us."

 —RŌSHI JOAN HALIFAX, founder and abbot of Upaya Zen Center

"There could not be a more urgent need for *Kinship Medicine*. The book's central message—that collective human wellness is inextricably linked to the health of the fellow beings with whom we share the planet—is an important contribution to contemporary discourse on topics ranging from climate change to economic inequality. Dr. Johnson argues that we are inherently part of the ecosystems we inhabit, and that we cannot be healthy when those ecosystems are sick and suffering. To the extent that we damage our biome, we also harm ourselves. Wendy makes these arguments cogently, and from the unique perspective of an experienced physician, activist, and public health expert able to limn connections between our individual health and the global forces that shape it."

 —DR. PAUL E. FARMER, cofounder of Partners In Health

"I devoured this book, hungry for its sumptuous wisdom on how we must come together in the soothing gardens of community if we are to nourish ourselves and the world. Dr. Wendy Johnson takes us to the cottonwoods and the coyotes and shows us the ecology cure to our individual and collective health. This book is a salve and a call to action."

—SONORA JHA, author of *The Laughter*

"A necessary book for our times. *Kinship Medicine* weaves Johnson's vast knowledge of human health from a physician's perspective with global history and philosophy, and her own life story on the land and with its creatures. Taken together, the book makes a brave argument for hope for a healthier future for us all—humans, other-than-human beings, and the planet—through connection and community. Despite the darkness of our current moment, the book leans into the light just ahead."

—ROBIN MCLEAN, author of *Pity the Beast*

"Dr. Wendy Johnson has written a needed prescription not just for better medicine but for a better life at both societal and individual levels. Take as directed. Please."

—WILLIAM DEBUYS, author *The Trail to Kanjiroba*

"*Kinship Medicine* is a wondrous journey through the systems of life, health, healing, and death from which we have become estranged, even in times when we think we know them all too well. As we build the communities we'll need to survive the climate crisis, it's good to know we'll be able to look to our side and see Wendy Johnson in the trenches, digging with us, and healing us when we blister."

—RAJ PATEL, coauthor of *Inflamed*

"Dr. Wendy Johnson makes an elegant, intelligent, and heartfelt case for new ways of thinking about humanity's place on Earth. Aspirational and celebratory, but also clear-eyed and historically informed, *Kinship Medicine* revolves around a central point: ideas matter, and the creation of a sustainable future urgently requires us to challenge some of the most basic cultural and philosophical assumptions of the Western world."

—FRANK HUYLER, author of *White Hot Light* and *The Blood of Strangers*

"*Kinship Medicine* explores modern America's destructive disconnection to the depth, breadth, and essential importance of the natural world. As Americans born into 'ecological catastrophe,' Johnson urges us to overcome our fog of amnesia and recognize our need to be in relationship with our environment. To regain our own health, we must commit to the care and protection of every species, every ecosystem. Johnson maps a way forward to a sustainable, hopeful future with wise and compassionate directives, encouraging us to step into wild places, engage in community-building partnerships and endeavors, and be informed and inspiring activists in the creation of a better world."

 —LESLEY POLING-KEMPES, author of *Ladies of the Canyons*

KINSHIP MEDICINE

KINSHIP MEDICINE

CULTIVATING INTERDEPENDENCE TO HEAL THE EARTH AND OURSELVES

Wendy Johnson, MD, MPH

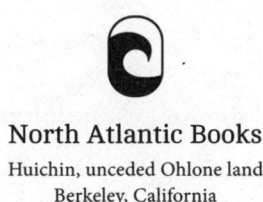

North Atlantic Books
Huichin, unceded Ohlone land
Berkeley, California

"Before the Flood" from THE PUPIL by W.S. Merwin, copyright © 2001 by W.S. Merlin. Used by permission of Alfred A. Knopf, an imprint of Knopf Doubleday Publishing Group, a division of Penguin Random House LLC. All rights reserved.

North Atlantic Books
Huichin, unceded Ohlone land
2526 Martin Luther King Jr Way
Berkeley, CA 94704 USA
www.northatlanticbooks.com

Cover art © Knstart Studio & aves
via Adobe Stock
Cover design by Jasmine Hromjak
Book design by Happenstance Type-O-Rama

Printed in Canada

Kinship Medicine: Cultivating Interdependence to Heal the Earth and Ourselves is sponsored and published by North Atlantic Books, an educational nonprofit that collaborates with partners to develop cross-cultural perspectives; nurture holistic views of art, science, the humanities, and healing; and seed personal and global transformation by publishing work on the relationship of body, spirit, and nature.

North Atlantic Books's publications are distributed to the US trade and internationally by Penguin Random House Publisher Services. For further information, visit our website at www.northatlanticbooks.com.

The authorized representative in the EU for product safety and compliance is Eucomply OÜ, Pärnu mnt 139b-14, 11317 Tallinn, Estonia, hello@eucompliancepartner.com, +33757690241.

Library of Congress Cataloging-in-Publication Data

Names: Johnson, Wendy (Wendy Lynn), author.
Title: Kinship medicine : cultivating interdependence to heal the Earth and ourselves / Wendy Johnson MD MPH.
Description: Huichin, unceded Ohlone land, Berkeley, California : North Atlantic Books, [2025] | Includes bibliographical references and index. | Summary: "For fans of Braiding Sweetgrass, The Future We Choose, and The Blue Zones, a book about the effect our relationship to nature has on our well-being and health"— Provided by publisher.
Identifiers: LCCN 2024048670 (print) | LCCN 2024048671 (ebook) | ISBN 9798889842736 (paperback) | ISBN 9798889842743 (epub)
Subjects: LCSH: Nature—Psychological aspects. | Environmental psychology. | Human ecology.
Classification: LCC BF353.5.N37 J64 2025 (print) | LCC BF353.5.N37 (ebook) | DDC 155.9/1—dc23/eng/20250326
LC record available at https://lccn.loc.gov/2024048670
LC ebook record available at https://lccn.loc.gov/2024048671

This book includes recycled material and material from well-managed forests.

1 2 3 4 5 6 7 8 9 MARQUIS 30 29 28 27 26 25

Contents

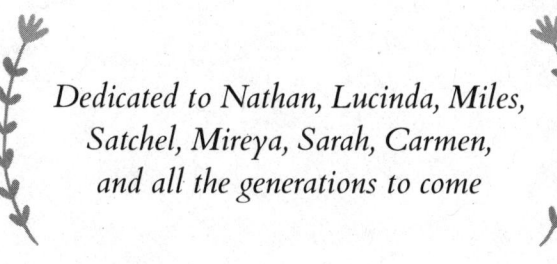

*Dedicated to Nathan, Lucinda, Miles,
Satchel, Mireya, Sarah, Carmen,
and all the generations to come*

I wanted us to start then
nobody will believe us
I said that we are building
an ark because the rains
are coming and that was true
nobody ever believed
we would build an ark there
nobody would believe
that the waters were coming

—*W. S. Merwin, "Before the Flood"*

Introduction
Out of the Fire

Man is the most insane species. He worships an invisible
God and destroys a visible Nature, unaware that this
Nature he's destroying is this God he's worshiping.

—HUBERT REEVES

New Mexicans know that spring is the season of strong winds, which often come on unpredictably. We humans may curse the dust storms that leave a thin film of dirt on every surface and the tumbleweeds that accumulate in our yards, but the ravens love those blustery days. From my back porch I've watched them frolic in the currents, like skilled surfers riding wave after wave. Three or four dark acrobats dancing in the gusts, circling back, catching the best ride, playing and performing for each other.

The weather in spring 2022 evoked the opposite of playfulness for most New Mexicans. Each day, powerful squalls sucked precious molecules of water from the air and land, fanning the flames that were burning up homelands of neighbors and loved ones just a few miles away. From early April until mid-June, I felt a sting of grief and trepidation in my heart every time I woke to the sound of the winds

---

A version of this chapter appeared in *Hinterland* no. 14, Climate Writing Special, January 2024.

battering my metal roof or saw the unbroken expanse of blue sky portending another rainless day. During the commute to and from my job as medical director of a community clinic in Santa Fe, I could see gray-black smoke billowing and spilling over the high mountain ridges of the Sangre de Cristos. Each day, my level of worry for patients, coworkers, and friends who lived in the path of the fire grew, matching the size of the clouds on the horizon.

Almost 900,000 acres of my drought-starved state burned that year, more than three times the annual average. Twenty-one large wildfires beleaguered the land and trees and wildlife and people. One of those fires was the most destructive in the state's history. The Hermits Peak/Calf Canyon fire indiscriminately devoured ponderosa pine forests, ancestral ranches, and critical watersheds. Another fire in the southern part of the state burned over 300,000 acres, about 500 square miles, and was the second largest in the state's history. Even as the monsoon rains came unseasonably early and prodigiously, new fires were being reported through mid-June. Several weeks after the deluge started, the largest of the blazes still weren't fully contained and wouldn't be until August.

The Hermits Peak fire started as a controlled burn, deliberately set by the US Forest Service, trying to mitigate the damage done by years of fire suppression in this part of the country. Federal administrators from afar, most with little experience in the state, made the decision to go forward with the burn. A rumor circulated that on the fateful day the fire was set, a local resident went up the mountain and got on his knees in front of the official in charge, begging them to reconsider. A damning post-fire assessment revealed that the feds ignored the warnings of locals, failed to adequately consider weather forecasts, did not appreciate the severity of the drought, and neglected to have adequate safety measures in place in case things went awry.[1]

Just as locals had warned, a few days after the fire was set, an exceptionally windy day sent flames far beyond intended boundaries. Although firefighters temporarily wrestled the blaze into submission, another day of strong gusts acted like a giant bellows. The fire took advantage of parched landscape, tinder-dry from the worst drought in a millennium, to rage out of control.

A few miles to the north, a pile burn set by the Forest Service in January smoldered unseen beneath the leaf litter. Despite being seemingly extinguished, it endured through several snowstorms. In April, it finally erupted. Strong winds and ample dry fuel exposed by the snow's unseasonably early evaporation incited the embers into an inferno. The two fires combined, one from the south, one from the north, obliterating communities and ecosystems in their paths. The result was exactly the kind of catastrophe the prescribed burns were supposed to prevent. The Forest Service's early acknowledgment of causality and accompanying apology were weak balm for those who were destined to lose everything.

As a family physician, I am trained to look at a constellation of symptoms and diagnose the disease that produced them. As a professor of public health, I teach my students how to tease out the causes of causes. In my classes, I take them through an exercise to help them get at the sometimes-hidden roots of seemingly straightforward problems. Together we create elaborate conceptual diagrams, starting with the downstream problem written at the center of the whiteboard. At first, they are a bit flummoxed as they are not in the habit of this kind of free-form visual thinking. I reassure them by saying, "There are no wrong answers." A few students call out the most obvious reasons for the problem we choose—for example, high maternal mortality rates are linked to poor access to healthcare. With some prodding, we get to the population-level factors, like racism and inequality. I challenge them to keep asking why; what caused that to happen, and then again, what were the contributing factors? When they think they've come to the beginning of the causal thread, I encourage them to probe yet again: What led to that outcome or circumstance?

In the case of the Hermits Peak fire, New Mexicans are outraged about the most proximal cause—a decision by federal agents of the US Forest Service to start a prescribed burn during our famously windy spring in epic drought conditions.

The strong desire to assign blame immediately led to class-action lawsuits and online petitions to terminate those responsible. The Forest Service responded by halting prescribed burns for a few weeks to reevaluate their policies. It seems a closed case, but if we draw the thread out a little further: Who else might be complicit? How many different overlapping lines of both inaction and action led to this tragedy?

The first humans who lived here used regular seasonal burns to keep forests in check and nurture an environment better for the edible plants and animals on which they depended. Tewa and Keres people, the original human inhabitants of the place I now call my home, whose descendants live nearby to this day in their ancestral villages, carefully cultivated this land for millennia before Europeans arrived. They domesticated food crops, irrigated fields, and nurtured an optimal environment for wild animals and plants they needed for sustenance. As such, humans acted as a "keystone species" much the same way beavers do when they build dams—altering the landscape so they might thrive, but also benefiting many other creatures and fostering biodiversity. They let natural fires burn, or even set them intentionally, to eliminate excess brush before it could accumulate and give rise to more intense and destructive conflagrations. The people indigenous to this place learned to interact with natural systems and adapted them to their benefit in a cooperative, symbiotic ecosystem.

In the late 1500s, when the Spanish conquistadors came to New Mexico searching for gold and silver and new territories to expand their empire, they came with their own technologies and ideas. The existing irrigation systems of Indigenous people were expanded to meet the needs of a growing population. An extensive network of hand-excavated ditches, called acequias, transformed the desert into fertile ranch lands. Domesticated sheep, goats, and cattle replaced their wild relatives. European settlers throughout the West dammed rivers and transformed canyons into reservoirs, often flooding out Indigenous communities and ecosystems.

The settlers were determined to make the land safe for their farms and families by subduing perceived threats. As colonial settlements grew, spreading to almost every corner of the mountain and desert landscape, the seasonal burns had to be stopped before they could threaten new villages and ranches. Without these small cleansing and renewing fires, the brush and deadfall accumulated. Over decades, the forest became overgrown and tinder-dry, like a bomb waiting for a spark to ignite. Many years of fire suppression combined with the worst drought in twelve centuries and an intensely windy and dry spring created the perfect conditions for the historic Hermits Peak/ Calf Canyon fire.

What of the causes of the drought itself? It might seem obvious to conclude that drought stems from a lack of water, but here again the real reasons are complicated. Total precipitation in New Mexico hasn't changed dramatically in recent decades, but temperatures have increased significantly, so more is falling as rain rather than snow. Warmer weather means that even when we do get good snows in the mountains, much of it evaporates before it can feed the rivers and refill reservoirs. What little snowpack that remains in the mountains by March or April melts far more quickly than it did just a few years ago, as higher altitudes are warming at an even greater rate than lower ones. Rather than streams recharging slowly over months, the spring runoff is often over in just a few weeks, and the water doesn't stay around long enough to seep into the ground. As the earth becomes desiccated, the plants that help hold on to water die off, and the soil becomes increasingly impervious to moisture. Like a dried-out sponge, the earth then requires more sustained and steadier hydration to penetrate and renew it.

I have seen these dramatic shifts in just the past decade of living here. A few years ago, the acequia behind my home was dry for two springs in a row. No one could remember that happening before. The cottonwoods are dying all up and down the valley. What if one day, the acequia never runs again? Will my water rights, entitling me to draw two acre-feet from the ditch to irrigate my land, become a quaint and faded vestige of a previous time, like an old photograph of a long-passed ancestor?

Our ecosystems are constantly changing, and for thousands of years now, humans have played a central role. All these changes affect nature's resilience and ability to respond to fluctuations in weather over time, but the relatively recent overarching influence of global warming and climate change dwarfs them all.

Going back to our web of causes, we've already uncovered many culprits for the unthinkable fire season of 2022, from fire-suppression practices to the loss of Indigenous knowledge, to overpopulation and colonization, to drought and high winds, to global warming and climate change. Let's keep going and ask: What is causing climate change itself? In my class, I teach students to back up the assumptions they make in their conceptual diagrams with research. In this case the evidence is clear and overwhelming. The United Nations puts it succinctly: "Today we are experiencing unprecedented rapid warming from human activities, primarily due to burning fossil fuels that generate greenhouse gas emissions." That statement implicates most of us, certainly those of us living above the median income brackets in rich countries of the world. As the old Pogo cartoon said, "We have met the enemy and he is us." In our personal lives we try to mitigate the harm we knowingly do every day. We recycle and drive or fly less and eat local organic foods, but we know in our hearts that these individual changes won't push the needle of climate change too much. Every shift we feel empowered to make is offset by the much-larger engine that powers society at large. We feel trapped in a system that doesn't allow sustainable choices most of the time. It's like trying to bail out the *Titanic* using a one-gallon bucket. Even millions of us making those small individual choices won't stave off the inevitable.

During my public health classes at the University of Washington, when I challenge students to think about the upstream factors that led to the problem we're considering, I also ask them to think about downstream consequences. In the case of the Hermits Peak/Calf Canyon fire, of course there are the immediate health effects I saw in my clinic every day—the exacerbations of asthma, emphysema, and heart disease. We know also that air pollution kills insidiously, causing heart attacks, strokes, and even dementia years later. The immediate displacement of people and loss of homes will result in physical and mental health struggles for generations of affected families. And of course, there's the degradation of precious wild places, the destruction of watersheds, the loss of so much wildlife, and the decimation of habitats vital for keystone species.

In the exam room, I started routinely asking patients from the burned area about the ways they were affected. A middle-aged woman who looked older than her years despite her jet-black hair paused for a long time before she answered. It was as if she had not considered how the events might impact her health. At first, she seemed relieved, telling me that her family's ancestral home sitting at the far end of Gallinas Canyon was spared while all the homes and forest around it were burned to the ground. Then she sat silently for another moment and started to tear up. She finally said softly, "The winds pushed the fire so far down into the valleys and canyons. It looks like giant claw marks etched into the hills. How can we return when so much of what made our home is gone?"

Ecologists agree that these forests will never really come back, at least not in their former state. The conditions that nurtured the ponderosa pines and spruce and aspens, the elk and cougar and bear, the trout and cottontails and owls, simply no longer exist. Humans were also a part of these ecosystems, and although they might return to the scorched land, the fires threaten to eliminate an increasingly rare way of life. Families on the destroyed homesteads and ranches trace their origins back generations, to the time when Spanish settlers intermarried with Indigenous people and transformed the desert into pastures and fields. In the villages of Mora County, nestled in the valleys and foothills of the Sangre de Cristo mountains, it's not uncommon to find a family living in a home built by their great-grandfather. The culture that grew up in northern New Mexico is heavily influenced by the ways Native Americans still live on this land, infused with the idea that humans and nature are co-dependent and in kinship with each other.

Herman Lujan and his wife, Lorraine, lived on the same land in much the same way their ancestors have lived for centuries. For all of his eighty years, Herman depended on the forests to sustain him. He sold timber for firewood and to build fences and barns. He grazed his herd of thirty cattle on the same land that was grazed by his father's and grandfather's herds. For years Herman had been nurturing some larger trees to selectively log, but the fires reduced Herman's ranch to charred ashes. It was little solace for the Lujans to find their home and a bit of surrounding land in the small town of Cleveland was spared, when everything that once sustained their family went up in smoke. For a few months, they tried to keep the cattle alive with trucked-in hay on the few acres around their home, but eventually they sold the whole herd.[2]

Herman's son-in-law, George Trujillo, is a Mora County commissioner. He and his family depended on the forest for their economic, physical, and mental well-being. When he talks about life before the catastrophe, he remembers trips up to the family cabin high in the mountains and the sense of peace and wholeness he felt just relaxing and watching wildlife and trees. "Now when I go up there I just cry and come right back down. People don't understand what we lost," he says. Things have not gotten better in months since the fire—"on a daily basis we are going through the same nightmare." Herman and Lorraine have rarely left their house in two years. The floods that followed washed out many of the forest roads, including those to the old family ranch. Unable to access his land, Herman sold off all his sawmill, logging, and butchering equipment. George was recently diagnosed with PTSD.

The ecosystem that nourished generations of humans and wildlife will eventually come back in some form, but it's not likely that George or Herman will see its renewal in their lifetimes.[3] And whatever replaces the old way of life will likely bear little resemblance to the traditional community that nourished generations of Lujans and Trujillos. Although FEMA compensation funds have finally started to flow into the hands of residents, this too has caused problems.

According to Commissioner Trujillo, crime and domestic violence rates have soared and the drug problem in the county grew worse with the influx of millions of dollars. Flashy new sports cars, motorcycles, and ATVs abound on country roads where previously it was rare to see even a late-model pickup truck. Many longtime residents sold their ranches to wealthy out-of-staters with no historical connection to the land. "Mora is changed forever," George says, "the trees will grow back, but it will never be the same. How can the government make you whole for all the beauty that was lost?"

The fires are destroying a way of life that can teach us valuable lessons for the future. Many of us transplants are drawn to this place because we sense that a different kind of relationship with the natural world is possible. People who were born here use the archaic Spanish word *querencia* to describe their connection to the land. The word derives from *querer*, which means to love or desire. If you ask New Mexicans what querencia means, you'll get many answers, but all will convey a deep connection to the place where one is rooted, the home from which one draws strength. Paula Garcia, a resident of the town of Mora who had to evacuate her home, defined it for a *New York Times* reporter as "a cultural longing, a pull, that keeps us there."[4] The word acknowledges that we are part of the lands and the ecosystems that formed us.

Although it may be difficult to see in a moment of such devastating loss, there are bright spots and positive downstream effects of the fires as well. Tight-knit rural communities responded to the tragedy by opening their homes and farms to human and nonhuman refugees alike. A Facebook page set up to connect those affected by the fires to resources offered corrals for horses, pastures for livestock, and foster homes for family dogs and cats. A coworker of mine let relatives sleep in her bed for two months while she slept on the sofa of her one-bedroom apartment, and many families living in nearby Santa Fe, Taos, and Albuquerque provided refuge for second cousins and distant aunts and uncles. In the small New Mexico town of Las Vegas, restaurants handed out free meals to both fire refugees and firefighters.

The tradition of mutual support is withering in our modern society. Is it possible to learn something about resilience and survival from this sense of communal care common among northern New Mexicans?

Back in the classroom, I help students think visually about the public health problem they're tackling and build out conceptual diagrams until we've exhausted all the space on the whiteboard. When we finish, we stand back and take in the dense web of bubbles and arrows indicating the interplay between factors. The students look at the tangle and feel overwhelmed at first, but I ask them to squint their eyes a little and see if they can discern patterns, or what I call "linchpin" factors. Can they see common themes that run through the whole picture, or find a few factors that, if they were changed or addressed, would cause the whole house of cards to collapse? If they can do that, then they can trace the lines back and find something actionable, a way to intervene that is within their abilities to affect.

The experts tell us that global warming is no longer reversible. We are dangerously close to the tipping point, triggering a cascade of cataclysmic changes that will irrevocably alter the planet and create many more climate refugees from fires, floods, and droughts. If we cross these thresholds, access to food and water will be severely compromised for over half of the earth's human population. The news is filled with stories of famines, wars, and immigration crises directly attributable to climate change. If there's no way to alter some of these inevitable outcomes, if there is no linchpin that can be pulled to undo the effects of climate change, what then? How might we weather the impending storms?

I've seen the consequences of our disordered ways of living on our planet play out in the lives of my patients. The linchpin cause that emerges when I map a conceptual diagram of my patients' despair almost always comes down to dysfunctional relationships and a failure to recognize and honor our dependence on each other and the natural world. Our Western society is built on the myth that we are all separate individuals with complete control over our own destinies. Nothing could be farther from the truth.

The common lesson I've learned from my clinical practice, my years working in public health, and my time living in New Mexico is that when patients have strong relationships with their family or community and feel a deep connection to their place in the world, they have more resilience to come through the inevitable challenges and disasters. They may be altered or battered, but they are better prepared to recuperate, adapt, and renew. What's true of human communities is also true in nature.

During the past decade stewarding just the small patch of land around my house, I've experienced my share of grief. The wind fells a beloved tree, or the magpie babies I've watched all spring are wiped out by a gang of ravens on the first day they emerge from the nest. Most recently, I've been witness to the drought slowly strangling so much of what I've tried to nurture, despite my best efforts. But there are also abundant doses of joy and renewal. The dry windy spring that gave birth to the Hermits Peak fire was followed by a prodigious late summer monsoon. After frequent drenching, everything green rebounded in a riot of life reaffirmed, even some trees and plants that I thought were long gone. Half-dead cottonwoods sprang back to life, sending up a tangle of new shoots.

Since the dawn of the modern age centuries ago, humans have tried to bend Earth and her systems to our convenience. What if we went back to ancient ways and adapted to her instead, accepting some inevitable change even as we work to mitigate the worst harms of human carelessness? As I watch the ravens finding joy in the storms of spring, I wonder if we might also find beauty and even hope in our ever-changing world. Renewing our relationships, with both humans and other-than-humans, can provide us with the sustenance and resilience we'll require to get through the turbulent times to come.

Earth will survive. It will be reborn in ways none of us can imagine. Humans have the opportunity to be midwives to that rebirth. We can draw inspiration from examples past and present. We have choices and agency about how we will live on this Earth, but they have nothing to do with paper or plastic straws. We can choose to be in kinship with living things sharing our space and our moment in time. When we see our neighbors as loved ones and family, the struggle for survival becomes both grander and more personal. We fight harder for what we love. Our challenge is to relearn the truth that many of our ancestors knew instinctively—that the path to well-being for ourselves and the path back to a healthy natural world are inextricably intertwined.

This book is about both of those paths and the places where they merge and intersect. It's about how we humans might regain our keystone-species status. The first step on this road is a realization that our wellness depends on everything around us. It's impossible to travel either path, to our own restoration or to Earth's renewal, alone. Just like decreasing your personal carbon footprint won't by itself push the needle on global warming, the multi-billion-dollar wellness industry can't improve our collective human condition. We are embedded in the ecosystems we inhabit, and we can't be truly well as individuals when those ecosystems are sick and suffering.

The prevalent sense of separation from the natural world is so profound that when many of us hear the word *ecosystem*, we think of it as applying only to the nonhuman, non-human-made world. The word *ecology* similarly evokes an image of "natural" environments, unspoiled by humans. The root of both words, *eco-*, comes from the Greek *oikos*, which means home, or place to live. The term *ecology* was invented by German zoologist Ernst Haeckel in the late 1800s to mean the study of a place and all the relationships and systems contained therein, including those between individuals, between populations of different species, and even between the living things and the physical infrastructure. I use both these words to include all the relationships and environments in the overlapping biospheres we inhabit, whether human-made or not, living or inanimate, animal or plant or bacteria. The distinction between humans and nature is a false dichotomy. We are nature.

Our survival as a species depends on developing healthy, reciprocal relationships with the other living things around us. Fundamentally, this requires us to shed our human-centered way of viewing the world in favor of a "life-centered" frame. Philosopher Timothy Morton calls this "ecological thinking,"[5] and it's how we survived and thrived as a species up until a few thousand years ago. Darwin (or really Darwin's interpreters) understood only part of the story of evolution, boiling it down to "survival of the fittest." As biologist Lynn Margulis pointed out, collaboration, cooperation and symbiosis were likely more important for our species' evolutionary success than competition.[6]

On a superficial level, we might recognize that humans are part of a web of life and that all life is connected, but the reality is much more complicated. Our ecosystems are not really like webs, networks, circles, or even spirals. There's nothing linear about them. Morton uses the term *mesh*. Our biosphere is more like the most gigantic, tangled ball of thread imaginable, one that has strings of every size that you can see, but also invisible strands that we can't perceive. Somehow, every thread is connected to every other thread. Some of the connections are obvious, but most can't be known until a thread is cut or removed. Acknowledging this mesh of intricate connections and being aware that humans aren't the most important thread are the first revolutionary steps we all must take. Without this basic change in thinking, any adjustments of actions or behavior or systems will be insufficient and unsustainable.

Looking at problems in such a holistic, cohesive way takes practice and courage, especially in a world bent on separating, categorizing, atomizing, and creating silos. The Western education I received trains students to think in dichotomies of human versus nature, mind versus body, individual versus community. Specialists with narrow focus are rewarded more highly than generalists. Unlearning old ways and going against the trends of mainstream society takes time and a conviction that there must be a better way. The first step is to develop a soft focus and an awareness of things just beyond our perception, much like learning to look at those "magic eye" illustrations of the nineties. Patterns will reveal themselves only to those with the patience to see what is hidden in plain view. Correcting our course requires a new consciousness and a different way of relating to everything around us. Only then can we begin to envision the kind of society that centers and nurtures life in all its myriad forms.

This book is the culmination of a long journey. It includes things I've learned from many extraordinary individuals, starting in childhood. I had the extreme privilege of being raised by parents with a deep appreciation for nature, a strong sense of fairness, and lots of love for each other and us kids. From my Italian immigrant grandparents, I learned generosity and acceptance by watching the way they welcomed all into their boisterous home. When I came to early jobs in government and political organizing, I was searching for a way to apply the sense of justice and love for others that my parents and grandparents instilled in me. I quickly became disillusioned and sought out another path, choosing medical school because I believed that being a healer was all about compassion and care. Again I found little space for concerns of justice or even compassion on most days in the cutthroat environment of medicine, so I sought out oddball mentors who bucked the system.

I was lucky to find and befriend people like the late Dr. Paul Farmer, who dedicated his life to the Jesuit idea of "a preferential option for the poor," and Dr. Jack Geiger, one of the founders of the community health movement. Their lives exemplified the quote from Aboriginal Australian women activists of the 1970s who said, "If you have come here to help me, you are wasting your time. But if you have come because your liberation is bound up with mine, then let us work together." Mentors like these encouraged me to study public health, and that in turn led me to jobs and experiences across the globe and introduced me to many other friends, teachers, and patients who taught me about mutual aid, solidarity, and the real meaning of community.

Although my love of nature dates to annual family camping trips during my childhood, it was intensified by living in New Mexico, first in the late 1990s during my family medicine residency, and then since 2012 when I was invited back to my old residency clinic, this time as medical director. The sum of all these experiences and teachings has led me to the conclusions and ideas expressed in the following chapters. So let's start the story at the stop along this journey where I currently find myself, the community that has been my home ecosystem for the past decade.

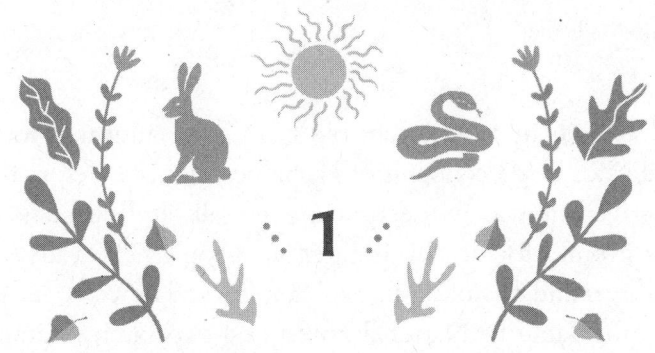

The Wild Tithe

I am not very hopeful about the Earth remaining as it was
when I was a child. It's already greatly changed. But I think
when we lose the connection with the natural world, we
tend to forget that we're animals, that we need the Earth.

—MARY OLIVER

A few years ago, I bought a house in a traditional agricultural village
of crumbling adobe homes on the outskirts of Santa Fe, New Mexico.
The half-wild valley is tucked into the foothills of the Sangre de Cristo
mountains, a spot called Chupadero, which literally means "the sucking place" in Spanish. Most nights, you can hear the coyotes' howls
echo down the arroyos. It seemed the perfect place for me, a family
physician who would rather be planting seedlings and pulling weeds
than treating illness or stitching wounds.

The home came with an acre and a half of orchard—some peach
and apple trees, a few drought-starved pears and plums—and a faded
whitewashed fence surrounding an overgrown vegetable garden. The

Versions of this chapter appeared in *Flyway Journal of Writing and Environment*,
Fall 2019, and also in *Chautauqua: Boundaries*, no. 17, Summer 2020.

house was built in 1993 on an old bean field cultivated for about a hundred years by descendants of Hispanic colonists. Before the Europeans arrived, it was winter grazing for elk and deer and a fertile hunting ground for nearby Indigenous people. The valley, with its seasonal river and mix of traditional families and newcomers, is nestled between the Santa Fe National Forest and two Native communities, the Tewa lands of Nambe and Tesuque.

The first Spanish settlers came to this high-desert valley around the mid-1800s and wasted no time building an irrigation system to give life to dreamed-of fields and pastures. Upon moving into the neighborhood, I became part of this centuries-old communal water sharing system, a so-called parciante, with rights and responsibilities to the land and the community. To attain this new title, I made my way to the New Mexico Office of the State Engineer for an appointment with Water Master Steve Maestas, an affable guy with an impressive shock of graying hair and matching almost-handlebar mustache/soul patch combo. I sat on the other side of his desk cluttered with documents and maps covering every surface, as he happily schooled this newbie on arcane New Mexico water laws. We traced the unbroken chain of water rights for my two acres back to 1876, from the Ortiz family who initially settled this valley down to me in 2015. My acequia is located in the Upper Rio Grande Region, District 6 Santa Fe, Nambe/Pojoaque/Tesuque Section. The water originates from the Rio en Medio above Aspen Meadows at about 10,000 feet altitude, splits off into a human-made canal for a mile or so, flows down the Sangre de Cristo mountains, through Pacheco Canyon in the Rio Chupadero, into our valley's Acequia Madre (colloquially called the main ditch), to Vicente Ortiz Acequia #2, and finally ending up irrigating the thirsty vegetable garden and orchard in my backyard.

As a parciante, I have the right to take two acre-feet from the acequia. It's a subjective measure, theoretically equal to the volume of water needed to flood my acreage one foot deep, which is only possible in a plentiful year. In drought years the ditch can be dry all season, and the gophers and grasses take advantage to claim it back as their own. The mayordomo and the commissioners of Las Acequias de Chupadero, chosen by all the parciantes, regulate the system. They are responsible for apportioning water fairly among the sixty or so parcels, over one hundred acres of gardens and fields.

My responsibilities as a parciante include contributing to the upkeep of the whole network, as well as caretaking my portion. In spring, we come together with our shovels and rakes and pruners for the lower ditch cleaning, "la limpieza." The limpieza is the great equalizer. All neighbors, rich and poor, are required to participate, all of us equally scratched and dirty after a day of battling the overgrown elms, Russian olives, and wild roses and raking the winter's detritus from the acequia floor. In fall, we all drive ten miles of steep, rutted roads, traveling together up into the mountains to maintain the origin of our Rio Chupadero—a cement and sandbag structure known as the splitting box—where it's cleaved from the more robust Rio en Medio. The diversion itself is an engineering marvel, a hand-excavated mountain-top channel traveling nearly a mile from the stronger flow of the Rio en Medio to the smaller Chupadero tributary through rough terrain strewn with granite boulders. In the 1870s, the two communities of Rio en Medio and Chupadero came together to build the diversion in a magnanimous display of cooperation and willingness to share a scarce resource, an early recognition of one of New Mexico's unofficial mottos: Water Is Life.

At least twice a year when we rake and dig and pull the worst of the weeds, we also share and connect and build relationships with each other. I ask about Jack's wife, who recently had a stroke, and we talk about organizing a meal train for them. David points out the best places to find the mountain porcini mushrooms, a delicacy called boletes, which emerge just a day or two after heavy fall monsoon rains. I learn from Frank the story of the roadside shrine, the descanso, a mile from the turnoff to our valley. It is lovingly maintained and updated every season in memory of his daughter, with red heart balloons for Valentine's Day, orange and black pumpkins for Halloween, a wreath and multicolored ornaments on Christmas.

"Somehow, I knew there was something wrong when she didn't come home that night, so I went out looking for her," he says. "I was the first to find her. She'd fallen asleep at the wheel and I found her there, almost home. There was nothing I could do." Even after ten years, we both tear up at the telling of the story.

Northern New Mexican acequia communities are distinctive for their lack of fences. Folks might have a coyote fence around a private patio, or a part of their land partitioned off for animals or pets, but it's rare to see a whole property fenced. The reasons are practical. We all are required to give access to the ditch for the mayordomo and the water commissioners to control the flows and fix problems, like collections of debris that can create dams after storms. The result is an open environment where we interact often with our neighbors, human and other-than-human alike. My dog-walk circuit climbs to hilltop views and descends through neighbors' yards where we greet my pup's neighborhood friends. The coyotes have their well-worn paths that wind around the river, through backyards, down arroyos; and the bears have their routes too, clearly remembering every fall where the best fruit trees and neighborhood beekeepers live. We see and hear the physical evidence every day of our interlacing lives: the nocturnal yelps and yowls, the tracks, the scat, the scattered compost, the piles of feathers or fur.

We don't often think about it, but our community is a throwback to earlier days when the commons was commonplace. Every community had shared space and activities that required all to cooperate for the common good, often for survival. Gary Snyder writes in his essay "The Place, The Region, and The Commons," "The commons is a curious and elegant social institution within which human beings once lived free political lives while weaving through natural systems. The commons is a level of organization that includes the nonhuman."[1] At one time, locally controlled common land was used for grazing, foraging, and hunting as well as irrigation. A few old Spanish land grants and tribal lands continue to be organized this way, as well as the many northern New Mexico villages that still maintain their acequia systems.

From the first days living here, my connection to this history, this ecosystem, this community felt familiar, like an old flannel shirt I had forgotten in the back of the closet. Growing up, my family moved every few years, an occupational hazard for my dad, who was a retail manager and always getting transferred to a new store. Three times in my school-age years, just after kindergarten, elementary school, and junior high, I was uprooted from my community of friends to an entirely foreign world. Each time, the only constant between my new and old lives was the outdoors, the woods and streams and trails always found near our homes, whether it was playing hide-and-seek in the yards of our urban Cleveland neighborhood, wandering the Metroparks near Toledo, or exploring riverbanks along the Sangamon in central Illinois. Weekends were spent in nature, often finding strays or attempting rescues of orphaned baby squirrels, rabbits, and birds. In the evenings I stayed up late under the covers, devouring stories like *Island of the Blue Dolphins* and *My Side of the Mountain* about children living alone in the wilderness. During long hikes with my black lab, Pepper, I found solace in the natural world when it seemed like the task of making a whole new set of human friends was too difficult.

After our last move, at the end of my freshman year of high school in 1981, I made a conscious decision to cultivate new friendships rather than just mope and mourn the friends I'd left behind. The resolve served me well throughout my life, as I continued to move often in my adulthood. I always managed to be that rare kind of nomad who is able to quickly learn about and absorb new cultures while creating deep connections to place and people. Over the past decades I've spent significant time in Chile, Chiapas, Mozambique, Seattle, and Cleveland and still maintain chosen family and friendships in all those places.

New Mexico made a significant impression on me the first time I lived here, in the late nineties during my residency in family medicine. It's rare, especially in the United States, to find a place where culture and history and the natural world are so completely woven into the fabric of daily life. In the years since my childhood immersions in nature, I've lived in several tight-knit communities, and I have also enjoyed many camping trips, hikes, rafting excursions, and other forays into the natural world, but until coming to this particular home, I never completely understood how the natural environment and a community of humans could be so intertwined and interdependent. After having lived all over the world, I returned to Santa Fe in 2012 to take a job as medical director in the same clinic where I completed my residency fifteen years before. I felt immediately re-welcomed into the community and rekindled old relationships.

During the first months in my new home, that old familiar connection to nature I had cultivated in childhood returned, but I sensed something new as well: an awareness of my reliance on the natural world and my responsibility to contribute something in return. I wanted to become useful to the land and hoped that we (the land and I) could develop a symbiotic relationship, along with the creatures that inhabited the space when I arrived, and who I hope will be here long after I am gone. I went about restoring the vegetable garden, reestablishing the compost pile, lovingly watering and pruning the fruit trees, shoring up the small pond, and setting out my beehives in a sunny meadow. Despite the century or so of cultivation, perhaps because of the proximity to the national forest, the wildness of this land was never completely subdued. An abundance of wildlife quickly appeared, much of it captured on trail cameras set out along the coyote highway that wends through the lower part of the yard, near the river, passing by my neighbor's chicken coop and my compost pile. The different markings and personalities among the coyote pack showed clearly on the videos and photos. There were the shy young ones, the bushy-tailed playful pair, and the big bold rust-colored one with the notched ear.

Although I welcomed the wild creatures and wanted to coexist, I was dismayed when I helplessly watched the magpies greedily gobble up ripe cherries on the uppermost branches that only they could reach, or when I discovered the beehives destroyed, with mounds of tiny bee corpses strewn across the yard after a midnight massacre-by-bear, or when I pulled up a carrot the size of my wrist only to find it was just a

nub, ragged with teeth-marks on the underside. A gopher had found
a snack conveniently protruding from the ceiling of his living room. I
felt a tinge of possessiveness the first settlers on this land must've felt, or
ranchers must feel today when they find a calf has been taken by a predator. These are my cherries—after all, what right does the magpie have?
The beehives I had worked so hard to nurture destroyed in an instant.
In years when drought threatens the fruit trees and makes me reconsider
the size of my vegetable garden, I get a small taste of the panic that must
have visited those early settlers who relied much more heavily on the
acequia. For them, dry seasons could mean starvation and death.

Then I remember, this land is not mine. I am no more the center of
it than the bear or the magpie. It was here for eons before I was born
and will be here after I am gone. In that long stretch of history, the idea
that one individual might "own" this spot of earth seems ridiculous. In
the blink of an eye I'll be just another pile of soil beneath the hillside.
The people native to this place have long understood this principle
and made offerings whenever taking something for their use, a wild
tithe, a gift ceded to our co-inhabitants. This portion of cherries or
carrots or honey is a tiny price to pay for living in a vibrant ecosystem. Besides, everyone does their part: the magpies eat the insects that
otherwise devour the crops, the gophers aerate the land, and I'm sure
the bears are important somehow too, even if I can't see it, and I can
still mourn the dead bees.

I employ a few nonviolent conflict resolution methods on my
small patchwork of wildness and cultivation: an electric fence surrounding the hives, some buried chicken wire encircling the garden,
a little netting over the berry bushes. Still, the coyotes peruse the
compost pile buffet almost nightly, the gophers run roughshod under
the wildflower meadow, leaving an odd mound of dirt in their wake,
the salamanders and bull snakes and pack rats and owls play out their
dance of predator and prey, but now I offer my contribution to the
animals who share this space more freely than before. I think of the
cherries on the uppermost branches, or the honey from the hive, or
the few nibbled carrots, as my wild tithe. I understand our mutually

beneficial unspoken agreement, and I no longer curse the pecked peach. Although I am still startled when the earwigs scuttle from the pit.

This dance of reciprocity with my wild neighbors has led to relationships that benefit us both. One summer, I noticed on the wildlife cameras that one of the coyote compost-pile regulars was startlingly threadbare. I had seen him before, walking through my backyard undaunted in the midmorning sun, or sauntering down the dirt road at dusk. He stood out, bigger than the rest, with a distinctive red-brown coat the color of rusty barbed wire and a notched right ear, the remnant of a battle with a neighbor's Chow-mix rescue. But now he looked like an exotic hairless dog with a few remaining tufts of fur jutting out at odd angles. As a physician, my mind jumped into diagnosis and treatment mode. Surely, he had mange. Can coyotes get mange? Can they get better on their own? How could I help him? Google and a call to a veterinarian friend taught me that coyotes do indeed get mange and that it can be fatal if it weakens their immune system enough or lasts into winter when a thick coat is essential for survival. The treatment is simple—an anti-parasitic drug called ivermectin. My ingenious delivery method: smear small amounts on stale bread and bury it in the compost. The wildlife camera tracked the treatment progress, and Red, as I had taken to calling him, was easy to spot with his distinctive markings. By November he was a new coyote, with a thick luxurious coat just like his brethren.

Not everyone has to become a coyote healer. But how might our relationship with the natural world shift if each of us asked "How can I be useful to the land?" rather than "How can the land (or my yard, or my garden) be useful to me?" Many of us feel a special connection to a piece of land—a childhood home, a park where we go for a walk every day, a farm or a wild place or a small patch of garden. Michelle Nijhuis writes, in a *New Yorker* article about the threats to public lands, that one could be connected to such places "by history, by heritage, by livelihood, by love."[2] I would add to that list "by intention." The core of our well-being is inextricably related to the health of the land, from the soil and the microbes to the grasses and the insects to the trees and the birds and the air. If we cultivate a desire to become native to the land and curb our arrogant assumptions that we can out-engineer nature, we might allow wild systems to rebalance—our own bodies included.

The Indigenous people who were here for millennia before the Europeans arrived had a starkly different relationship to the natural world that they carry forward to this day. They understood that humans are part of nature. Using keen empirical observations, honed and passed down meticulously for generations, Native peoples innately understood more about the ways of nature than Western scientific tools have taught us. The belief that humans were co-equal and co-dependent with all other living creatures was ingrained in myths and stories. In her book *Braiding Sweetgrass*, Dr. Robin Wall Kimmerer, a citizen of the Potawatomi Nation and plant ecologist, retells the creation story of her people when Skywoman came down to Earth from the stars as the first human being. She found a world filled with strange creatures and was only able to survive and flourish because the animals adopted this foreigner, nurtured her, and showered her with gifts. She returned the favor with gifts of her own from the Skyworld, the plants and flowers and trees that nourished the animals on Earth. "Children hearing Skywoman's story from birth know in their bones the responsibility that flows between humans and Earth," Kimmerer writes.[3] Since intentionally choosing this patch of earth, I have begun to feel Skywoman's story in my bones. I choose to be in communion with this valley and the other inhabitants who share it with me, human and animal.

The places where one can practice the Skywoman ethos are rapidly disappearing. Our federally designated public lands may appear to be another kind of commons, but they are not controlled and managed by the local people who have the deepest connection to them. The habit of domination over the land, more often than not, dictates terms of use. Those who would exploit or extract are given priority for logging or grazing or mining, with decisions made by authorities who may never set foot in the place. Although some areas are protected for wild things, even those are increasingly threatened. The boundaries encompassing these places are recognized only by humans, not by the coyotes or bears or mountain lions who know only their ancient territorial bioregions and can't read our signs.

Those of us who imagine that we can create a world separate from nature—subduing or eliminating its dangers, but still enjoying its pleasures when we desire—vastly overestimate our own cleverness. Nature is not so simple, easily dominated, or forgiving. Each environment's animals, plants, and even microbial species are part of an intricate choreography largely unnoticed by most humans. When a few of the dancers are removed, others overpopulate, and chaos and disequilibrium ensue. Science has yet to understand the ways all these moving parts work together. Often it is only after some piece is eliminated that we realize how essential it was to the healthy functioning of the whole system.

Here in northern New Mexico, despite being surrounded by so much natural beauty, our communities are often profoundly disconnected from their roots in the land. Several waves of colonization, gentrification, and historical violence in the form of dispossession of land, poverty, and destruction of communities have left their mark. New Mexico suffers from one of the highest rates of opioid overdose deaths in the country, and in my work as a family physician I treat many patients struggling with addiction. In their eyes, I see yearning for some lost connection they cannot name. They tell me their stories of trauma and how the drugs, mostly heroin, numb the pain of loss. But there are also stories of hope, like the young woman who was able to walk away from her addiction and rekindle the relationship with her parents. She found healing in the patch of earth her family has farmed for generations. She now lives with her young son in the house her grandfather built and is supported and cared for by her people. The patients who are most successful at overcoming their dependence on drugs are those able to reestablish their roots to culture, place, family, and community.

As I write this, it is late winter in my valley. The coyotes are celebrating the nascent spring with nightly choruses of high-pitched howls and excited barks. Although some of my neighbors are wondering if this long and snowy winter will ever end, the signs of rebirth are already there for the sharp-eyed. The flickers have begun advertising for a mate, drumming on the loudest things they can find, a hollow tree or, more frequently, my metal gutters. Soon the pond will thaw and the salamanders will start their mysterious migration from underground winter hollows to frigid underwater mud. The leaf buds are beginning to swell and the elms are blooming, offering a first taste of pollen to hungry awakening bees. When the ground thaws, I can harvest some of the sweet, overwintered carrots that the gophers may have overlooked. One can faintly detect a change in the air from the cold sterility of winter to fecund and floral scents of spring.

Living in this community has taught me to recognize these subtle signs, the nuanced offerings of nature in all its messy, intricate interconnectedness. I've come to understand viscerally that the health of our ecosystems is inextricably connected to our own individual and collective health. Throughout my life, I've experienced both connection with nature and connection with human communities, but this is the first time I've seen how the two can be integrated together, and how that integration might hold the key to solving many of the challenges to our environment and our health. Imagine if we prioritized restoring well-being to our environment as much as we prioritize our individual wellness, if we saw the two things as one and the same. At one time, almost all of us lived in communities with close ties to other humans and to nature, but now it's just a tiny percentage. If anything, current trends are making this way of living increasingly endangered, which is revealed clearly when we look at a snapshot of where *Homo sapiens* find ourselves this crucial moment in time.

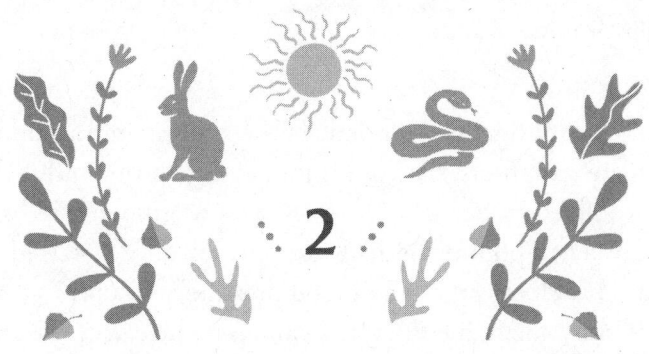

The Mess We're In

It's worse, much worse than you think.

—DAVID WALLACE-WELLS, OPENING LINES
FROM *THE UNINHABITABLE EARTH*

Robert's prodigious body was slumped dejectedly in the exam room chair. He looked up at me sheepishly as I entered, and I knew immediately he'd had another setback. We'd met over a year before, at his first appointment. He was in his late thirties, working as the manager of a local fast-food restaurant that didn't provide health insurance. Over the previous few years, nagging ailments had been increasingly plaguing him, until finally the headaches, weight gain, and fatigue became too much to ignore. Despite his fears of the expense and that he hadn't seen a doctor since childhood, he finally made his way into the clinic. On that first visit we diagnosed uncontrolled diabetes, dangerously high cholesterol, and high blood pressure. While this might have been devastating news for some, Robert took it as a challenge and changed everything about his lifestyle. He stopped smoking, improved his diet, and started exercising. He took all his medications every day. During those first few months we celebrated his successes together, and I thought he'd dodged the bullet, but then life intervened. Over the next six months, his wife left, he became a single parent raising two teenage daughters, he lost his job, and then one of his daughters became addicted to heroin. The stress was too much. He had gained back the twenty pounds he had lost plus ten more, started smoking again, and his blood sugar and blood pressure shot up.

As a family medicine doctor, I can empathize with Sisyphus. We have similarly impossible tasks. When I am alone with a patient in the exam room, I might feel like we've pushed the boulder almost to the top of the hill. We go through their medicines and make sure they understand the correct timing and dosages. We talk about their goals for diet and exercise. We discuss strategies to quit or cut down on harmful habits like smoking or drinking. We think together about how to address stress or depression in their life. I make sure they are up to date on all their immunizations and other preventive services like mammograms or the dreaded colonoscopy. Much of the time, we end the visit feeling pretty good about the plans we've created. But then my patients leave the idealized world of the doctor's office and go back into their daily lives, into our dysfunctional society, where they confront the intractable problems of racism, poverty, trauma, pollution, and the inability to meet basic human needs. Many suffer from lack of adequate housing, healthy foods, clean water, community relationships, opportunities for exercise, and connection with the natural world. These are the things we have come to call the "social determinants of health" but are mostly powerless to change from the vantage point of the healthcare system, even though they are arguably more important than individual biological factors. Between optimistic visits to the doctor's office, the boulder comes tumbling down, flattening my patients in the process.

Many of the places humans live aren't very conducive to optimizing our health. Some of us are engulfed in downright toxic environments—perhaps surrounded by trauma and abuse; or living alone and isolated from other humans; or exposed to ongoing assaults from poisons in the air, water, and even the food we eat; or separated from the healing power of the natural world. Like the proverbial frogs in a pot of water slowly brought to the boiling point, we often adjust to our harmful surroundings and don't realize how bad things are until it's too late. The killers are invisible and unrecognized, and once we feel the effects, the damage has been done. Far too little attention is given to these forces that determine much more about our well-being than individual genetics or biology.

Hierarchies and Health

All of us, no matter how rich we are or the color of our skin, suffer from the stressful effects of rampant racism and inequality. These forces break our communities apart and create divisions that make us distrustful and afraid of each other, adding to our sense of disconnection and isolation. Over the past fifty years, since the civil rights movement, we seem to be taking two steps forward and one step back in our progress toward becoming a more equitable society. Although we've addressed some of the most egregious encoded racist laws, like those permitting slavery and institutionalized segregation, the challenges that remain are pernicious. Our criminal justice system disproportionately targets people of color, and as a result, police violence is a leading cause of death for young Black men in the United States.[1] Black, Indigenous, and other people of color are incarcerated at five times the rate of whites in our state prisons. Health disparities lead to stark differences in life expectancies for both racial minorities and people living in poverty. The richest among us live almost fifteen years longer than the poorest on average, and white European Americans can expect to live up to seven years longer than Black Americans.

One might conclude that these inequities affect only those on the bottom rungs of the ladder, but the stress from living in a starkly unequal society affects us all, even those with higher incomes and lighter skin colors.[2] Societies with rampant inequality are more dangerous for everyone, with higher crime rates and fewer health and safety protections. Overall life expectancies at all income levels tend to decline in extremely inequitable countries. Over the past fifty years, the gap between the rich and poor has grown dramatically almost everywhere, with the United States now being the most unequal among all rich countries.

Where We Live

Over the last couple of centuries, our world has become increasingly urban. In the year 1800, 90 percent of the world's population lived in the countryside, mostly working in agriculture-related jobs. As of 2008, for the first time, a majority of people live in urban areas.[3] Many of those places are becoming so densely populated that outdated infrastructure is pushed beyond its limits, and resources like water and energy have to be carefully rationed. In 1950 Beijing had just 1.7 million inhabitants; by 2020 it had grown by more than tenfold to 18 million. Most of the world's great capitals have seen similar exponential growth.

The stress of living packed so tightly together with precarious access to resources takes its toll both physically and mentally. People in urban areas suffer from anxiety and depression at significantly higher rates than those residing in rural places.[4] More and more cities experience regular power blackouts and water shortages, compromising the health of their most vulnerable inhabitants. The World Health Organization (WHO) has declared the problem of urban pollution a "public health emergency," citing studies that show four out of five city dwellers are exposed to rates of air pollution that exceed WHO limits. In most cities it's the equivalent of smoking a pack of cigarettes every day.[5] Poor air quality not only causes respiratory illnesses but has been linked to strokes, heart disease, cancer, diabetes, obesity, depression, dementia, low birth weights, and even decreased cognitive abilities in young people. Globally, air pollution causes more than 8 million premature deaths per year.[6]

Dense urban areas with overstressed, and aging infrastructure are especially vulnerable to the effects of climate change. The unprecedented and lethal floods in Pakistan in 2022 resulted from a torrential monsoon season that delivered ten times more rain than average. Over 1,000 people died and the public services in Karachi, a city of 16 million, completely collapsed. Entire neighborhoods were submerged, displacing millions of people. In the aftermath of the floods, the WHO predicted the country would be ravaged by waves of epidemic infectious diseases like cholera, malaria, and dengue fever.[7] Closer to home in the same summer of 2022, the water system of Jackson, Mississippi, failed after heavy rains overwhelmed the city's water treatment facility. Over 150,000 people were without safe drinking water for a month and had no water at all for the better part of a week.[8] Every subsequent year now brings more extreme weather, causing death and destruction on a scale previously unthinkable. In 2024, Hurricane Helene wiped out entire towns and compromised vital infrastructure for months, affecting hundreds of thousands of people. By the time you read these words, another cataclysmic event (or many) will likely have occurred. Climate change and rising sea levels mean once-rare natural disasters are becoming commonplace. These "extreme weather events" are happening with such increasing magnitude and frequency that many go unnoticed by much of the world, especially when they happen outside wealthy countries. The September 2023 catastrophic floods in eastern Libya left over 15,000 dead or missing and another 40,000 homeless but went relatively unreported in the West.[9]

Even as cities have become overpopulated and unhealthier, rural areas have suffered in other ways. Mass migration to urban areas left small towns depopulated. Essential businesses like hospitals, pharmacies, schools, and grocery stores closed, job growth stagnated. In both southern Ohio and northern New Mexico where I have worked, dollar stores proliferate, taking the place of grocery, pharmacy, and general store. They offer almost exclusively the processed foods and high-calorie drinks that drive obesity and diabetes pandemics. In the United States, rural areas tend to have higher rates of poverty, higher rates of uninsurance, and less access to healthcare, healthy foods, or opportunities for exercise. Despite beautiful surroundings, those who live "out in the country" are often still disconnected from nature due to lack of public lands, poverty, and systems that favor processed foods over locally grown products. Over time, old traditions and connections to the land are forgotten. One shocking example of this phenomenon was related to me by colleagues who work in a food bank in southern Ohio. They noted that their clients consistently prefer potato flakes from a box over actual potatoes. When asked why, one person stated that she didn't know how to prepare the whole potatoes, so they usually just rotted untouched.

Our Exploding Numbers

The existential crisis of our time, climate change, is directly related to the immense extraction of fossil fuels necessary to satisfy growing needs of an exploding world population. There are more of us living on Earth than ever before, and our appetites are growing as well. It took about 127 years for world population to double from 1 billion in 1800 to 2 billion in 1927, but only 47 years to double again to 4 billion in 1974. We reached 8 billion in 2022. Although that growth rate is slowing somewhat, another billion people are added to the population every 12–15 years, or about 80 million new humans per year, all of them needing at minimum basic necessities like food, water, and housing.[10] From Aristotle to Malthus to Paul Ehrlich, experts and thinkers have debated how many people the earth can accommodate, the so-called carrying capacity of our biosphere, with estimates ranging from 4 to 16 billion people. The direst predictions about overpopulation leading to widespread famine and devastation have not yet come to fruition, mostly due to advances in food and energy production, but those technologies have come at a high price.

Since trees became an important resource for fuel, buildings, and paper, almost half of Earth's forests have been cut down. Most of those that remain are hollow facsimiles of the rich biodiversity held by old-growth forests they replaced. Because of climate change, drought, and increased wildfire threats, global rates of deforestation are skyrocketing in recent years. Over 75 percent of land on Earth and two-thirds of ocean areas have been significantly altered by human activities.[11] About 70 percent of accessible freshwater has been commandeered to grow crops and livestock to feed the growing numbers of us.[12] Scant space or resources are left for the rest of the living beings with which we share the planet. We are crowding them out of existence.

While the numbers of human beings have been increasing dramatically, the numbers of most other living things, especially those we don't actively cultivate for food, have precipitously declined. As *Homo sapiens* claim more and more of Earth's surface for our own purposes, we are pushing all the other creatures to the margins. Biologists believe that the sixth great mass extinction event since the beginning of life on Earth is in full swing, with the loss of up to 200 species every day.[13] That rate is tens or even hundreds of times the normal background loss expected without the inordinate effects of human activity. Up to one million plant and animal species are predicted to become extinct in the coming decades. Perhaps even more dramatic than the number of extinctions is the sheer loss of total numbers of other life-forms and overall biodiversity. In the past fifty years, populations of wildlife have fallen by over 70 percent and continue to precipitously decline. Humans and domesticated livestock now account for 96 percent of the total biomass of mammals by weight, with wild animals making up only 4 percent.[14] Wild areas and habitat are diminishing both from direct human occupation for homes and agriculture, and the effects of global warming.

We are already experiencing the consequences of climate change on human health. Volatile storms, destructive wildfires, and epic droughts and deluges have become the norm. I drove through Lake Charles, Louisiana, after the first of two "100-year" hurricanes hit in 2020 and was shocked at the level of devastation: houses blown off their foundations, almost every building with a damaged roof and windows, and most ominous of all, it looked like winter, even though it was late August, because the winds had blown all the leaves off the trees. The mayor and residents lamented that they were forgotten in the crush of other natural disasters and the coronavirus pandemic, and it seems they were right. Five years after those storms, the majority-Black city with a poverty rate of over 20 percent has yet to recover. Many homes are still uninhabitable, and some residents have been living for years without running water or functional roofs.

There is no doubt among the scientific community: the world is getting hotter, weather events are more severe, and humankind is to blame. It's a simple and inescapable equation. Society's dependence on fossil fuels puts massive amounts of carbon into the atmosphere, while at the same time, the capacity of "carbon sinks," forests and grasslands and oceans, to remove the carbon is rapidly diminishing. Since Bill McKibben wrote *The End of Nature* in 1989, first sounding an urgent alarm, scores of books have carefully documented the effects of climate change on humans and the planet. They are wide-ranging and encompass almost every facet of our lives, from where and how we live to what we eat and drink to the air we breathe. The likelihood of war and conflict will increase dramatically, cities will flood or become too hot for humans, and as a result, the World Bank predicts, there will be up to 200 million climate refugees by 2050—just 25 years from now. The last dramatic global climate change event happened 100 million years ago and took place over 40,000 years. Scientists say that this change may be an even greater shift over a much shorter time, only 150 years or so. The challenge is immense, and time is running out.[15]

But Aren't Humans Healthier Now Than Ever?

Less biodiversity or some bad weather might not seem like a significant threat to human health. After all, modern medicine and public health interventions have contributed to extending our life expectancy since the early 1900s from less than fifty years to well into our seventies today. Food and energy production innovations have touched almost everyone on the globe and made life better for most of us than it was for our great-great-grandparents. Advances in medicine and public health have subdued most common infectious diseases. Technology seems to save us every time. Even a devastating global pandemic is far less deadly, on a per capita basis, than a similar one was a hundred years ago. Thanks to science, effective treatments and vaccines were rapidly developed during the COVID-19 pandemic, saving thousands of lives. But how much better if the specter of global pandemics wasn't such a huge threat in the first place?

Over the past few decades, a balance has shifted; technological advances have been increasingly inadequate in mitigating the harms coming from unhealthy surroundings. In the United States, life expectancy has mostly stagnated since 2010, and even had its biggest decline in 2020. While many rich countries saw life expectancies dip in 2014–15 due to an unusually harsh flu season that winter, the UK and US have flatlined since. Researchers point to various causes including "deaths of despair" from overdose, alcoholism, and suicide; rising rates of cardiovascular and other chronic diseases; and more recently, the coronavirus pandemic shaved a few more years off average lifespans. All these different causes of illness and death have one thing in common—their root causes come from the environment. They can all be seen as the effects of living in degraded ecosystems. The most important reason our ecosystems are suffering is the dysfunctional relationship between the human-made environment—our modern human societies and cultures—and the natural environment. A more accurate moniker might be "deaths of disconnection."

Our healthcare system is woefully unprepared to address maladies that come from the conditions of our lives. The disciplines of clinical medicine and even public health tend to focus mostly on individual biological traits and behaviors. Healthcare providers talk to patients about eating a better diet, exercising more, and quitting bad habits like smoking, drinking, and drug use. In some cases, we even have pills or shots that treat unhealthy behaviors, like those to help people stop smoking, curb appetites, or treat dependence on opioids. But for most patients, these fixes are nothing but temporary fingers in the dam—short-term Band-Aids that don't address root causes. Some people may be able to improve a few behaviors and get a little healthier, but for many, sooner or later, the overwhelming negative influences of their daily surroundings will win the day.

As I see my patients, I think how much easier my job would be if we all lived in homes that were safe and free from contamination, in places where community and family relationships were fostered and encouraged, and where the natural world was integrated into daily lives. After a long day in the clinic, pushing the boulder up the hill with my patients, I take one last look at my electronic medical record inbox. The requests have been piling up throughout the day, and I try to triage and respond to the most urgent ones that can't wait until tomorrow. Even so, I find myself staying an hour or two after clinic most days and still carrying my patients' worries with me as I get into my car and drive the fifteen miles back to my home in a tight-knit rural community on the outskirts of Santa Fe. I wonder about patients like Robert, and what his life may have been like if he had not deferred seeking healthcare so long because of the cost, if he had assurance of a job or a basic income, safe housing, and access to mental health care.

I turn off the highway onto a winding country road lined with wildflowers in late summer. The arroyos, mountains, and spectacular Santa Fe sunsets form a soothing backdrop. As I drive deeper into the countryside, I feel a visceral change. The stress of the day melts away. I recognize how privileged I am to have this refuge, a place where the natural world is a constant presence, where I know all my neighbors and a sense of community is pervasive. I wonder how I might do this journey in reverse and bring nature and community back into the lives of my patients and our whole society. But to get back to a place of connection, it's important to understand how we came to this dark place of polarization and isolation.

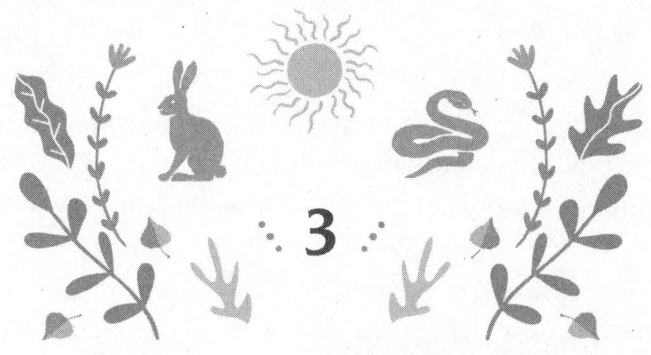

How Did We Get Here?

Nature as family became nature as machine, and our non-human relatives, our teachers, became mere objects for consumption.

—ROBIN WALL KIMMERER

Ute Mountain rises over the desert plain like a whale breaching from calm waters. Hundreds of millions of years ago, this expanse on the northern border of New Mexico was in fact a shallow sea. The mountains encircling it erupted as volcanos millions of years later during the last ice age, and a mere few millennia ago, the glaciers receded and a desert slowly formed.[1] The word *desert* is often synonymous with *barren* in our modern lexicon, but the dusty landscape provides a rich and nourishing environment for many species that have evolved together to live here.

The mountain gets its current name from the Ute people, who have lived here for eons. Before the Spanish invaded in the mid-1500s, the Utes shared this place with other living beings in relationships that were symbiotic and interdependent. The area inhabited by the Utes was immense, comprising what is now part or all of Utah, Nevada,

Arizona, Wyoming, Colorado, and northern New Mexico. The Utes organized themselves into twelve distinct groups, each with their own habits and systems, but united by a common language and cultural values.

Who Belongs to the Land

The band of Utes who once freely roamed the Rio Grande and San Luis Valleys in northern New Mexico and southern Colorado are known as the Caputa. They moved across the landscape in very specific rhythms, according to the season and their needs. The word *nomadic* may connote homelessness and aimless wandering, but in the case of almost all nomadic peoples, each journey had a specific purpose. Like other migratory species, the Utes optimized their relationships to the earth, traveling ancient routes they knew by heart, always at home in the thousands of acres that comprised their well-worn pathways.[2] They adapted to changes in climate and environment, altering the timing or locations of their movements to match the pulse and patterns of Earth herself. Their trails were later used by successive waves of colonists and today are often overlaid by highways and interstates. The idea of land as property was unknown to the first human inhabitants of America, but there was a commonly recognized reciprocal bond that each community had with their ancestral territory and migratory routes.

In the centuries since the Spanish irrevocably disrupted these ancient practices, the Utes' territory has been claimed successively by many interlopers. The first would-be conquistadores arrived from the south, claiming the land for the Spanish Crown. They brought diseases like smallpox that devastated the Ute people, and their livestock destroyed crops and food plants that were critical for survival.[3] The Utes tried to adapt to this new ecology as settlers and fur traders encroached into their lands. They adopted some commercial ways of the invaders and traded for horses, food, and guns. Like the northern Plains Indians, the Utes became expert riders.

In 1806, two centuries after Utes' first encounters with Europeans, the settler president Thomas Jefferson sent Zebulon Pike to explore the newly acquired Louisiana Purchase, which extended to the eastern portion of what is now Colorado. Pike claimed and renamed one of the Ute people's most sacred places, Tava Mountain, now known as Pike's Peak. Colorado and New Mexico were still claimed by the Spanish Crown and, later, the independent Mexican government, which handed out huge land grants to its citizens in the early nineteenth century. Stories of the rich abundance of timber and wildlife and newly discovered gold and silver in the San Juan Mountains attracted more European settlers by the late 1800s.[4] President Jefferson himself recognized that these early seekers of wealth were "the overture to . . . American settlement of the West."[5]

In 1848 the United States seized the entirety of Ute territory as spoils for winning the Mexican-American War. The Utes never ceded any of their lands nor accepted conquest by Spain, Mexico, or the United States. Over the years, the Ute people resorted to violent means to defend their homeland out of desperation as they watched settlers take the best rangeland and decimate populations of buffalo and beaver. In 1849 the US Army responded to the Utes' last-ditch efforts to protect their way of life. Acting on a desire to make the western frontier safe for white settlers by finally subduing the Indians, the US Army destroyed fifty Ute lodges, important communal buildings that housed families and served as cultural gathering places. Faced with an overwhelming and cruel adversary, the Utes were coerced into signing a treaty recognizing the sovereignty of the United States. The forced "agreement" defined boundaries of their territory and compelled them to "cease the roving and rambling habits which have hitherto marked them as a people" in favor of "cultivating the soil" and confining themselves strictly "to their allocated lands."[6] Subsequent treaties in the late 1800s continued to whittle away at Ute territory while bestowing lucrative mining rights or title to rich agricultural lands upon white pioneers.

Encroachments on Indigenous stewardship of the land continued apace with the Homestead Act of 1862, which granted 160 acres of land to any man who would promise to live on it and "improve" it, displacing Indigenous people from over 270 million acres—400,000 square miles—across the western US. In a final blow, the Allotment Act of the late 1800s sought to definitively sever Native Americans' relationship to their homelands. The law authorized the US government to divide up land held communally by tribes and allocate it instead to individual tribal members and families who would be encouraged to adopt European-style farming practices and customs and "assume a capitalist and proprietary relationship with property."[7] In this way, it was hoped that Indigenous traditions would eventually die out and Native Americans would be fully assimilated. Over time, much of the allotted land fell into non-Indigenous hands, and only a small fraction is still held today by the original families. In just a few hundred years, the Southern Utes went from ranging freely in an area of over 100 million acres to a reservation of just 681,000 acres in southwestern Colorado.

Nature for Human Consumption

A portion of historical Ute territory surrounding the mountain now named for their people was declared a national monument by President Barack Obama in 2013. I have come here to take a remote hike just after monsoon storms passed through and drenched the parched earth, giving the terrain a vibrant glow. A rutted dirt road encircles the mountain and provides great views of the Rio Grande Gorge, which now sports an array of temporary waterfalls as the deluge washes through the arroyos and down into the river below.

Among the hierarchy of public lands designations, a national monument is somewhat protected, but humans can still enter to drive the roads or to hike, hunt, fish, and camp. "Existing rights" to the land before it was a designated monument are also recognized, including any oil or gas leases, livestock grazing, or private property easements that predated the designation. Ute Mountain is the centerpiece that marks the northern edge of the Rio Grande del Norte National

Monument, an area that stretches along the Rio Grande River from the Colorado border to Taos Pueblo some forty miles to the south. The mountain is still a sacred site for the local Indigenous people, including the Tiwa of Taos Pueblo and the Utes.

To access the monument's entry gate, I drive on unpaved roads that wend through a patchwork of private ranches and homesteads. While ambling along one of these just outside the boundary of the public lands, I see a cleverly worded announcement on a fence surrounding a private ranch.

The warning advises pet owners that traps and snares are present in the area to "capture harmful animals." Best to keep your dog on a short leash. The ominous sign goes on to inform that like the nearby national monument, the traps and "the animals captured in them are the property of the United States Government" and that "tampering with these devices or the sign is a Federal offense." Unfortunately, coyotes and bobcats, the likely targets of these traps, can't read the signs, nor can they know the boundaries between public lands where they may be somewhat protected and private ranches where they are fair game.

The entity responsible for posting the sign is the United States Department of Agriculture, Animal and Plant Health Inspection Service, Animal Damage Control, better known by its Orwellian nickname "Wildlife Services." The agency is charged with ensuring that your hamburger ends up on your plate and not in the mouth of a hungry wolf. Their mission, as stated on their official website, "is to provide Federal leadership and expertise to resolve wildlife conflicts to allow people and wildlife to coexist." Their primary method of resolving conflicts is extermination, and disputes with over two million mammals and fifteen million birds have been settled this way since 2000, by the agency's own estimates.[8] This is akin to General Custer advertising his services as "conflict management" with Native Americans.

The agency's origins date back to the decade just after Custer's last stand, in the late 1800s, when the US government was bringing all its resources to bear in its quest for Manifest Destiny, the idea that European settler dominance over this land was a God-given right. The goal was to conquer the West and claim the land for white settlement based on farming, ranching, and mining. This endeavor required eliminating not only the Indians but also the bison, coyotes, wolves, bears, and cougars—anything that stood in the way of making the wilderness "safe" for mining gold and silver, grazing cattle and sheep, and planting fields of wheat and corn. The elimination of the buffalo was especially insidious, tied directly to the genocide of Indigenous peoples, the Utes among them, who depended on buffalo as an important source of food, clothing and shelter, and a touchstone of their culture.

The mission of the agency has not changed substantially since the 1800s: it still exists to make the land safe for private business interests. Today, the perceived threat is mostly from the wilderness itself, specifically from predators. In the eyes of many ranchers, the West will not be conquered until their cattle can graze for almost nothing on public lands purged of all risk. Any rancher can claim compensation from the government for livestock taken by wild animals and can also call on Wildlife Services to eliminate the offending predators, hence the signs like the one I saw. Ranchers want to have their steak and eat it too by availing themselves of the bounty of the wilderness while being protected from its uncertainties and dangers, even though there is no strong evidence that the practice of predator elimination actually helps livestock in the long run.

Take the case of the lowly coyote, perhaps the animal most reviled by ranchers and subsequently the most massacred—now that wolves have been mostly extirpated. The US government kills about 70,000 coyotes per year, at a cost of about $20 million of our tax dollars. They use traps and poisons that often ensnare non-targeted wildlife; they use expensive aerial hunts. Another 300,000 coyotes per year are killed in private hunting contests. All of this is done in the name of protecting ranchers' livelihoods, but there exists almost no connection between coyotes and significant loss of livestock. Recent research done by Wildlife Services itself shows that killing coyotes can create the opposite of the intended result. The coyotes adjust to the disruptions in their packs by having larger litters at an earlier age, a kind of natural balance reset button. Wantonly erasing the perceived threat of coyotes has proven counterproductive over time, as eradicating wolves and buffalo—both keystone species—did before them. The systematic elimination of wolves and cougars in the last century was a major contributor to the coyote population explosion in the first place. In most cases, when humans question nature's intelligence and assume to know better, the ensuing unintended consequences are far worse than the original "problem."

Over the course of 500 years or so, this land has gone from being a rich and biodiverse ecosystem where humans coexisted as equals with other animals to one that is dominated and exploited by humans. Even the national monument designation is primarily intended to serve human needs for recreation and resource extraction. If the needs of the ecosystem as a whole are perceived to conflict with those of the humans, the humans always win out. This abbreviated history of inhabitation and conquest in one corner of the earth is not exceptional. Stories like this one are common in every part of the globe. In just the past few hundred years, almost everywhere on the planet, *Homo sapiens*' relationship to our environment changed dramatically from one based in interdependence, integration, and symbiosis to one of conquest, dominance and exploitation. How did things go so awry?

The First 90,000 Years

Humans, in our current iteration of *Homo sapiens*, have been kicking around on Earth for at least 100,000 years. For more than 90 percent of that time, it never occurred to our forebears that they weren't part of nature. They viewed other living things around them as allies or competitors, predators or prey, but also as brothers and sisters—as kin.

Sometime about 5,000 to 10,000 years ago, in a dramatic change, our ancestors shifted from being mostly hunter-gatherers to becoming nearly full-time farmers. The transformation was gradual, taking thousands of years. Even the term *hunter-gather* now seems outdated, implying that in pre-agriculture times, people simply happened upon what they needed to survive and lived completely at the mercy of their surroundings. Recent research confirms that humans had been shaping their environment for a very long time before taking to the plow. Like beavers and other keystone species, *Homo sapiens* and other early humans created conditions that made it easier to hunt or forage, made homes safer, and ensured nourishment throughout the year. The environment around them was cultivated to favor certain species over others. Useful plants were carefully observed and given what they needed to thrive, transplanted to more convenient locales, or even cultivated and domesticated to produce more prodigiously. Pasturelands were created from forests to give the large grazers humans depended on for food and hides their preferred open grasslands. Indigenous people invented permaculture.

Pre-agriculture humans saw themselves in a reciprocal relationship with nature, using their intellect and tools to shape the environment around them. Their methods were mostly symbiotic and nurturing rather than dominating and destructive; and the effects were so seamlessly integrated that they mostly went unrecognized by anthropologists and archaeologists until recently. All over the world, Ingenious technologies used by the first peoples are being rediscovered, but much has been lost. The plagues and following genocides that decimated New World inhabitants after contact with Europeans wiped out much cultural knowledge about living embedded in nature, expertise that we desperately need today.

In school, I learned that the first human inhabitants of the Americas were called Indians, that they lived in teepees in close-knit familial groups, they hunted for food, had few possessions, and existed almost magically in an undisturbed wilderness. Many carry this image of the noble savage, shaped in elementary school. It is almost entirely wrong.

The original peoples of the Americas lived in all kinds of communities from small family camps to large, densely organized cities. Their ruins can still be seen in the southwestern United States, Mexico, and

Central and South America. The largest of these so far discovered in the United States lies in western Illinois, along the Mississippi River, and has been fully appreciated only in the last forty years. Its name, Cahokia, is taken from the people living there when French explorers first arrived, but the name, language, and culture of the people who built the settlement have been lost to history, as has the story of their city's rise and fall.

The inhabitants of Cahokia lived in a complex society centered around huge earthen mounds up to ten stories high topped with large wattle buildings. They produced copper, pottery, and tools from the local, highly prized "chert" stone, and they were part of an intricate trading relationship with other groups from the Great Lakes to the Gulf of Mexico. They had an advanced knowledge of astronomy and a calendar, reflected in arrangements of timber poles they erected to align with vernal and autumnal equinoxes. At its peak in the thirteenth century, the population of Cahokia rivaled that of contemporaneous London, with as many as 40,000 inhabitants. Archaeologists say that Cahokia was the most populated city in the Americas north of Mexico. The settlement had been abandoned for more than a century by the time French explorers happened upon it in the 1600s, and no one knows for sure what led to its demise. Theories range from depletion of the area's natural resources spurred by a sudden population boom, to flooding made more devastating by local deforestation. A deadly epidemic may have contributed as well, perhaps facilitated by the density and size of the population.[9]

All that remains to describe the lives of these and other first peoples are the oral histories passed down to their living descendants, the accounts of the European colonists and settlers, and the archaeological record. Even though journals and letters of foreign explorers are filtered through the cloudy lens of conquest and exploitation, their accounts are given the most weight in our history books. The picture handed down of pre-conquest America is limited because most first explorers did not imagine they had anything to learn from the Natives. Europeans did not see the "savages" they encountered as equals and were not particularly interested in habits or lifestyles of the peoples they encountered except as they could co-opt or exploit them. The relationship between the Native people of the Americas and their environment was so sophisticated and integrated that it was not recognized by the colonists as a system of natural resource management at all. It bore no relationship to the hard toil and backbreaking labor they associated with agricultural work in Europe. Still, they remarked on the manicured appearance of the forests, the carefully tended groves of fruit trees, and the abundance of the maize harvest, which seemed to produce more than their familiar European grains like wheat and barley.

In the scant few years before waves of epidemics stuck down much of the population, European explorers and colonists observed clusters of closely packed Native villages and noted how healthy and fit the people appeared. Giovanni da Verrazzano, the first explorer to embark on the shores of what we now call New England in 1523, remarked that the coastline was filled with smoke rising from bonfires and that the land was "densely populated." Verrazzano saw the Narragansett men as they paddled their canoes out to meet his ship and wrote that they were "as beautiful of stature and build as I can possibly describe." Accounts like these are repeated by early explorers throughout the Americas and the South Pacific.[10]

By the time Europeans started to create permanent settlements and interact more profoundly with the Indigenous peoples, disease had already wiped out much of the Native population. In many cases, the plagues spread far and wide after the first explorers returned home; subsequent settlers coming into areas Europeans had not yet reached encountered ghost towns where a thriving society had been just a decade or two before. Some scholars estimate that by 1700, up to 90 percent of the population of the original Americans succumbed to European diseases like smallpox, measles, and cholera. Europeans formed their ideas about what the culture of Indigenous American people was like based on the aftermath of a plague apocalypse.

The emerging picture of the First Americans before the plagues hit challenges almost everything taught in American elementary schools when I was growing up. The societies and cultures of those who lived in Cahokia, who built cities and towns in Chaco Canyon and Teotihuacan, Machu Picchu, and Tikal, and who first inhabited the New World, from the Inca to the Inuit, are much more complex than imagined by my grade school teachers. People were mostly healthy by all accounts, with life expectancies that rivaled those of the European invaders. They lived in egalitarian societies with sophisticated concepts of human and natural rights and a rule of law that allowed cooperation and freedom of movement across great distances. They had their own systems of science and medicine. In their cosmology, there was no division between mind and matter, body and spirit, nature and culture. The religion of First Americans was rooted in the natural world. The persistent myth that European settlers happened upon a vast, largely unpopulated and untouched wilderness and "civilized" it though grit, determination, and hard work hampers our ability to find a different kind of reciprocal relationship with the natural world in modern times. It feeds into a man-vs.-nature dichotomy and demands we take sides. In reality, the history of myriad different ways humans have found to live on Earth is much more complicated.

Although there were commonalities between the cultures of the Ute, the Narragansett, the Inuit, and the hundreds of other groups who inhabited the Americas before European contact, there were many more differences. Each culture embodied a unique way of living that was well adapted to their specific circumstances. Anthropologist Wade Davis coined the term *ethnosphere* to describe this totality of human knowledge gleaned throughout history. He describes it as

> *a cultural web of life . . . the sum total of all thoughts and dreams, myths, intuitions and inspirations brought into being by the human imagination since the dawn of consciousness. The ethnosphere is humanity's great legacy. It is the product of our dreams, the embodiment of our hopes, the symbol of all that we are and all that we have created as a wildly inquisitive and astonishingly adaptive species.*[11]

Throughout human history, there were once thousands and thousands of answers to the question "How should we live on this earth?" Now only a narrow few dominate popular thinking. How did our collective imaginations get so constrained?

How Humanity Got Stuck

Conventional wisdom tells us that the agricultural revolution is to blame for our current predicament. For the first few millennia of human experimentation with what we now call agriculture, harvests were small and seasonal, supplementing hunting and foraging. Almost everyone continued living close to the land, developing vast empiric knowledge of their natural environment. Over time, the story goes, dependence on agriculture became increasingly necessary and central. It took so much labor to tend fields that little time was left for other activities. Populations grew quickly, fueled by new abundance, and so much space was occupied by the crops and livestock that other species previously hunted and foraged became sparse or displaced. Our species' deep knowledge of the rhythms of the natural world began to atrophy.

As agriculture became more important, communities grew larger and larger, thereby necessitating even more reliance on farming and the surpluses it could provide. Technology and tools grew more sophisticated. Supplemental subsistence plots that would feed a family or small community gradually morphed into large feudal plantations. Abundant harvests led to problems that hunter-gatherers never encountered. Large stores of grains needed to be guarded, and larger cities required leaders to coordinate labor and distribution of the surpluses. The support required for such complex operations included many specialized professions, from warriors to blacksmiths. Farming larger tracts of land required not only better tools but also cheap, exploited labor. A hierarchy emerged, and the world suddenly became divided into leaders and workers—a few kings, priests, and lords on one side, and many peasants, artisans and slaves on the other.

A plethora of scholarly books makes this progression seem inevitable. Hierarchies and militaries and oppression are simply the price we must pay for civilization. New discoveries in archaeology, however, are casting some doubt on the old received wisdom. David Graeber and David Wengrow explain in *The Dawn of Everything* that large cities dependent on agriculture existed without much evidence of hierarchies or a ruling class. If we go back as little as a few thousand years to North America or Crete or Mesopotamia or Mexico, we find examples of advanced and flourishing civilizations, full of art and culture but devoid of the hallmarks denoting divisions between humans into elite and oppressed classes. This new evidence calls into question the inevitability of the current forms of organizing human society. For reasons hotly debated by historians, those other models were either abandoned or conquered, and our extremely hierarchal modern world came into being. It took no time for a whole underpinning of religion and philosophy to develop around this new world order, justifying its existence.

God and Man

Before the dawn of large-scale agriculture, leadership was often rooted in generosity. A chief showed care for his community by sharing resources, often in rituals and ceremonies, like the potlatch of the Pacific Northwest peoples. In post-agriculture communities, leaders came to think of themselves like the queen bee in a beehive—indispensable. They believed, and convinced their followers, that the community would cease to exist without them, and therefore they deserved preferential treatment and protection. In this way, class divisions emerged, along with ideologies and myths to justify them. Philosophers and religious leaders were only too happy to oblige, currying favor with the rulers.

The first spiritual beliefs held that humans were an integral, co-equal part of nature, rather than above, superior, authoritatively ruling over her. These theologies were firmly rooted in nature and intimately connected to the local landscape. Spirits were associated with specific trees, plants, animals, and even inanimate objects. Natural phenomena were explained through the actions of spiritual beings. If a living creature was taken or destroyed, its spirit was acknowledged and thanked. All of life was held as equally sacred. This way of thinking is embedded in the languages and cultures of Indigenous people, like the Ashaninka living the Peruvian Amazon. Their name for themselves encompasses not only their community of humans but also their other-than-human family, including other species they consider kin. Similar beliefs are still held today by Indigenous groups all over the globe.

As the agricultural revolution gained steam, different ideologies and religions were necessary to justify the new order of things. Animist beliefs of hunter-gatherers slowly gave way to polytheist religions of the early agriculture period and finally to large monotheist religions that hold sway over much of the world today. Gods of the first polytheistic religions promised humans special advantages over their brethren through sufficient devotion. People asked the gods for abundant harvests, good weather, or the birth of healthy children. When those things happened, it was proof the new gods were superior to the old ones. When things went badly, the fault lay with devotees for failing to offer sufficient prayer and sacrifices. Polytheism was mutable and flexible at first, swallowing up and adapting local gods of conquered cultures when necessary. The spirits of animist religions existed alongside or were incorporated into polytheist beliefs. Over time they fell out of favor and became less potent as control of the natural world and the necessity of establishing and maintaining hierarchal relationships among humans became more critical.[12]

The shift from nature-based religions to beliefs centered on relationships and hierarchies became more pronounced in classical antiquity as the earliest forms of Judeo-Christianity. Soon monotheism took hold in the form of Judaism and Christianity, followed quickly by the growth of Islam. Even more than the polytheistic beliefs they replaced, these religions emphasized hierarchy, putting man at the top of the societal pyramid. They justified monarchy and slavery, ushering man from his position of communion with wilderness to domination over it. Oppression and coercion were the primary tools used by monotheists to convince nonbelieving pagans to give up their faith in a world imbued with spirits everywhere in favor of one omnipotent god.

All these elements are contained within the biblical creation myth. God begins by making the earth and the living things inhabiting it. The culmination of his masterpiece is the creation of Adam in his own image. The entire world is created for Adam's comfort and pleasure, including Eve. God tells Adam that he is the master of this world and gives him the task of naming all the living things. The fall of man from paradise comes because Eve is too interested and engaged with the natural world in the form of the apple tree and a snake. Her curiosity overtakes her obedience to God. The devil is represented as an animal. God is supernatural, above nature, not a part of it. The messages are clear.

Western Science Turns the Universe into a Machine

Religion may have taken the first blow at severing the symbiotic relationship between humans and nature, but Western philosophy and science soon joined the fray. As far back as 350 CE, Aristotle described a natural order that put man at the top of a pyramid of life, ruling over nature. He saw a hierarchy with plants at the lowest level, possessing only "life," animals next, possessing life and perception, and finally humans on the top with life, perception, and "logos," meaning the capacity for rational thought, moral reasoning, and language. In *Politics*, he wrote, "Plants are for the sake of animals and . . . other animals are for the sake of human beings."

Philosophers Francis Bacon and René Descartes solidified the Western schism between man and nature in the early seventeenth century. Descartes's ideas gave birth to the Western scientific method, reducing all knowledge to what could be objectively measured and laying the groundwork for the Age of Enlightenment that followed. Descartes described animals as automatons: machines incapable of thought, reason, or emotion, acting solely in response to outside stimuli. He thought the human body functioned like a machine as well, but distinguished by "a mind which is capable of rational thought without reference to any passion," setting humankind apart from other living things. Descartes promised we could become "masters and possessors of nature," and with Bacon, believed that all the workings of the natural world could be unlocked through reasoning and empirical observation. Bacon went even further, believing that "nature, to be commanded, must be obeyed," acknowledging that man had to understand the "laws of nature" before he could dominate it. Presaging animal cruelty in the name of scientific experimentation, Bacon advocated "putting nature on the rack . . . as torture may compel an unwilling witness to reveal what he has been concealing."[13]

Descartes, Bacon, and their disciples in Western philosophy thought the world was divided into matter and the material world on one hand, and the mind or conscious thought on the other. In Cartesian metaphysics, only humans possessed a mind capable of self-consciousness or a soul, and these qualities were separate from the functions and sensations of the body, which operated in mechanical ways that could be discerned by applying empirical methods. The human body itself and everything else in the world of nature was fair game for experimentation, exploitation, and domination.

The Enlightenment unlocked an era of abundant scientific discovery but also extreme social stratification. The idea that human bodies were autonomous machines whose secrets could be revealed by close observation began to grow in Western cultures. Though the soul was beyond the reach of empirical assessment, those advocating the new philosophy still made judgments about the nature of the soul and God. They felt that animals were clearly a separate class of being from Man because they lacked souls and couldn't think. Women were somewhere in between, possessing souls, but inferior ones. In procreation, the soul was said to be located in the sperm, with the womb serving only as a protective vessel. It was believed by many that during the final resurrection of Man, all humans would be reborn as men, as this was the version of humankind closest to God.

Slavery, Genocide, and Colonialism

Making the leap from "humans are closer to God than animals" to "humans are not animals" to "some humans are closer to God than others" and finally to "some humans are more like animals than others" did not take long. The Western belief that some people were less human than others has been used to justify oppression, slavery, and genocide for millennia.

The practice of large-scale slavery is believed to have started around 3,000 years ago, about the same time intensive labor was required for larger agricultural outputs. Slave and beast were equal in the eyes of Roman law, both treated as property of their owner. The penalty was the same if you killed a man's slave or his goat. Aristotle observed of slaves: "Animals do not apprehend reason, but obey their instincts. Even so, there is little divergence in the way they are used, both of them (slave and domesticated animals) provide bodily assistance in satisfying essential needs." He argued that slavery is an innate personal characteristic, that some are destined to become slaves because of their "slavish nature" while free people have a "free nature."[14]

Male European colonists and explorers took reassurance in Western religion and philosophy of their God-given superiority, and even their duty, to lead and dominate those of other races. They found justification for cruelty and oppression in the Christian Bible but also used Western science to confirm their beliefs that other races weren't fully human. When early European explorers in West Africa first encountered Africans and also great apes like chimpanzees, they remarked on the similarities between the two, even postulating sexual relationships occurred between them. Their journals record this as an empirical, even scientific, observation. Throughout the nineteenth century,

Europeans used now-discredited "scientific" techniques, like measuring human skulls, to conclude that darker-skinned humans were an altogether different species.[15] Africans were situated somewhere between beasts and humans on the scala naturae, or the Great Chain of Being, a supposedly God-given ranking of all forms of life first proposed by Aristotle and commonly accepted by early colonists.[16]

Feminist scholar Donna Haraway coined the term *plantationocene* for the latter part of the agricultural age, when farms were industrialized and became monocrop plantations necessitating the exploitation of labor and the earth's resources. Slavery was a crucial component in building the planation-based economy of the early United States. In that era, those who were enslaved were considered no different from livestock, and slave-masters believed them incapable of moral reasoning or higher thought. Frederick Douglass described his experience being the subject of a slave auction: "We were all ranked together in valuation, men and women, young and old, married and single, were ranked with horses, sheep and swine. There were horses and men, cattle and women, pigs and children, all holding the same rank in the scale of being, and were all subjected to the same narrow examination."[17]

Similarly, many of the first European settlers in the Americas viewed the Indigenous people they encountered as not quite human, and the Catholic Church was only too happy to oblige early colonists and homesteaders by sanctioning the colonial project as "God's will." The so-called doctrine of discovery was laid out in a series of fifteenth-century papal bulls that maintained the superiority of Christians over nonbelieving heathens in Africa, Asia, Oceania, and the Americas. The doctrine held that any European explorer had the right to claim newly "discovered" territories in the name of Christian monarchs back home, even if they were already inhabited by non-Christian peoples. The decrees explicitly condoned slavery and even genocide of Native peoples in the name of spreading Catholicism and Western culture throughout the globe. The doctrine of discovery inspired the American ideas behind Manifest Destiny and the Monroe Doctrine of the 1800s. Reference to it is even enshrined in US legal discourse in the form of an 1823 Supreme Court decision against the rights of Indigenous people to own and control land. The chief justice at the time wrote for an unanimous court "that the principle of discovery gave European nations an absolute right to New World lands," over and above the rights of Native peoples.[18] The ruling held that the original inhabitants of the land might have the right to occupy but could not sell or transfer the land because they did not "own" it. That right was reserved exclusively for European conquerors.

Eradicating Dangerous Ideas

The ancient worldview of man's integration with the natural world and the sacredness of all things didn't succumb easily to these new philosophies. In many instances the old world view had to be violently overthrown and stamped out, both in the colonies and at home. The Enlightenment overlapped with the height of a witch-hunting craze in both Europe and North America. Religion and science combined forces to eradicate dangerous beliefs held mostly by women who refused to subjugate themselves to a God that didn't believe they were fully human. The witch hunts reflected the era's struggle between faith in the natural world and faith in the word of a Christian God who demanded obedience and complete submission.

Witch hunters believed they could find objective evidence of witchcraft, like special markings or telltale behaviors. Prominent scientists joined with church leaders to rout out and punish practitioners of what was considered the devil's magic. William Harvey, an English physician famous for the first accurate description of blood circulation, lent his own expertise to scientifically discerning the identity of witches. By carefully examining subjects (in one case by dissecting a toad, the animal companion of an accused woman), he empirically determined the status of women in question in at least two documented cases (in both, he decreed the women were not witches).[19]

Over the course of 300 hundred years, from the fifteenth to the eighteenth century, up to 100,000 people, mostly women, were killed in witch hunts and trials. In some villages of northern Italy and Germany, the entire population of women was nearly wiped out. Many of the murdered were midwives and doctors, using healing methods that had been developed by empirical observation over centuries. As women were deemed lesser creatures, incapable of rational thought, they were immediately suspect if they claimed to be using their intellect or espoused views at odds with local religious leaders.

The colonial project and the witch trials both had their roots in Christian supremacist ideas of man's domination over nature. Cotton Mather, the leader of the Salem witch hunts, believed that Christian New Englanders had settled in the devil's territory and had a duty to civilize and sanctify it by strictly adhering to God's will. He believed the practice of witchcraft, as he defined it, was contrary to what God intended, even though most of those labeled witches identified themselves as Christian. In the minds of those who hunted and killed witches, they were eradicating a dangerous sect who refused to submit to the authority of God and chose instead to follow evil spirits, echoing the original sin of Eve in the Garden of Eden. The supposed witches were suspect because of their kinship with animal "familiars" and their reliance on natural medicines and practices rather than on prayer and piousness. Because of their threatening idolatrous worship of nature, they had to be eliminated.

My own family tree includes both witch hunters and witches. I am distantly related to Cotton Mather on one side, and my Italian grandmother hails from Friuli, the part of Italy made up of isolated Alpine villages that was heavily affected by the witch hunts. Visiting my Friulian cousins and wandering through the cemetery where gravestones display just a few surnames of the families who have inhabited this valley for hundreds of years, I have wondered about the lives and fates of my great-great-grandmothers. I am literally the descendant of the witches who survived, but also of the witch hunters.

Two Anthropocentric Views

Over the past 500 years, the modern world has been heavily shaped by contemporary Western European thought and practices, and Western culture now dominates much of the globe. Although most disavow extreme expression of these ideas like witch hunts or slavery or Indigenous genocide, almost every aspect of society worldwide is heavily influenced by the religious and philosophical beliefs that gave rise to these atrocities. The anthropocentric worldview is so ingrained, and humankind's disassociation from nature is so complete, that it goes relatively unnoticed. Debates about climate change, environmental conservation, and the future of the environment are imbued with the assumption that humans are the central concern. The dominant worldview is segregated into the domain of humans, devoid of nature, and the domain of nature, devoid of humans. This binary stalemate asks us to choose between two possible futures—one that prioritizes the interests of humans versus the health of the environment, or vice versa, as if these two are at odds with each other. In fact, the two futures are inextricably entwined.

For many centuries, the resources of the natural world seemed so vast that we never worried about exhausting them. Even today, die-hard believers in human superiority are confident that our God-given intellectual prowess will allow us to find technological fixes to our environmental problems without having to curtail our destructive habits. These people diminish the value of nature or reduce it to a mere commodity for human consumption. They believe that preserving a few examples of endangered species in zoos or parks is sufficient. When he was running for governor of California in 1966, Ronald Reagan expressed that mindset in a speech to logging industry leaders: "I mean, if you've looked at a hundred thousand acres or so of trees—you know, a tree is a tree, how many more do you need to look at?"

On the other hand, some extreme conservationists swing the pendulum in the opposite direction, yearning to return to a pristine human-free environment that never existed. The myth of pre-1492 America as an untouched, largely unpopulated "virgin" wilderness, and a desire to return to this imagined past, has influenced the environmental movement, leading to another untenable binary outcome.

Our public lands today are overlaid with a patchwork of different designations, each with their own regulations governing official uses, almost all human-centered. Historically, these areas have been managed by bureaucrats with little personal connection to the land they oversee. The goal is to maximize "ecosystem services" while balancing the need for resources with the need to enjoy nature for its own sake. Some tracts are held to be more pristine, but in most of these, the land is managed so that the "wilderness" is tamed and made safe for humans by eliminating predators or building roads. Ironically, many of those areas, like our national parks, are sacred places where Native peoples previously lived in close relationship with nature. To create the managed and controlled wilderness we enjoy today, original peoples were dispossessed of their homelands. Very few public lands are managed in a way that gives top priority to wildlife and natural ecosystems.

The struggle is mostly between two extreme ideas at polar opposite ends of anthropocentrism. In both cases, our habit of domination over the land dictates uses. At one end is exploiting or extracting to benefit humans without regard to nature; on much of our public land, priority is given to logging or grazing or mining. On the other side is protecting some special islands expressly for wild things, excluding all but a few humans—a kind of colonized wilderness where any trace of the first humans to live there as a part of nature has been erased. Neither of these ways of relating to nature is sustainable.

Shifting Lifestyles in an Instant

Five hundred years is a brief moment in evolutionary terms, yet in that short time, almost everything about the way we live, the food we eat, and our relationships to other humans, to the land, to animals, and to the natural world has changed dramatically. The shift into a fully agrarian-dependent society took us millennia. The leap from agrarian-based economies, with most people living in rural societies interdependent with the natural word, to highly socially stratified industrialized economies with most living in massive cities, happened in a blink of Gaia's eye.

For thousands of years before the modern era, we evolved symbiotically with the other living things around us: the microbes, plants, and animals we interacted with every day. We lived close to the earth: eating a varied diet, following seasonal biorhythms and sleep cycles, and moving our bodies by walking, running, squatting, stretching, for much of the day. We lived in interdependent, tight-knit communities and families. The relationships we forged to other humans and the natural world around us continued throughout most of our lives and were critical to our well-being.

Although the roots of our disassociation from nature may go back thousands of years, most of us descended from ancestors who remained close to the land throughout the agricultural revolution. Go back three or four generations and you will almost certainly find an ancestor who subsisted on a combination of farming and foraging, who intimately knew her surroundings, the names of hundreds of plants and animals, and which ones were good for food and which for medicine.

My grandmother and grandfather told me stories of living from the land in this way in the places they grew up in the early twentieth century, the Italian Alps and the Adriatic coast. They gathered mushrooms, plants, frogs and fish; their families tended extensive gardens and kept some goats and chickens. When they emigrated from Italy to New York, they imported that lifestyle as well. My grandfather hunted deer and foraged for mushrooms to supplement the food he grew on his small farm (now a car dealership on the outskirts of Buffalo, New York). My grandmother made dandelion salads from the "weeds" in their yard.

The life most of us live bears little resemblance to our ancestors from just a few generations ago. We get less sleep, eat an unhealthier diet, and if we exercise at all, it's relegated to a couple of hours per week at the gym. Many of us live in relative isolation, fewer and fewer people in larger and larger homes. The number of meaningful relationships we have with friends and family has dwindled, and our communities are less cohesive. In exchange for nearly constant exposure to nature, we are now bombarded daily with hundreds of human-made substances—air and water pollution, food additives, cosmetics, pesticides, drugs, cleaning agents—most developed within just the past fifty years or so, many with unknown long-term effects on our biology.

Fueled by twin engines of colonialism and capitalism combined with the Western world's entrenched ideologies that humans are superior beings, we seem unstoppable. Industrialization accelerated our ability to exploit the earth through increasingly rapacious and destructive extractive industries for fossil fuels, timber, and other necessities. We gained the ability to move around the globe in a matter of hours or days rather than years or decades. A few generations ago, most of our ancestors lived their entire lives within a few miles of their birthplace. Now we are genetic amalgams from all over the world. My genes come from Sweden, Italy, Germany, and England. Before the nineteenth century, each of those ancestors grew up and grew old in a reciprocal relationship with their local environment. In my life, I've lived in New York, Michigan, Illinois, Ohio, Chile, Mozambique, Seattle, and New Mexico. Deep connections with land and place have been severed for most of us, with profound but largely unacknowledged impacts on our bodies and psyche.

A New Way Forward

We are at a crossroads. Will humankind continue down a path of separation from nature, of domination and destruction, or will we harness our intelligence toward finding new ways of achieving integration, reciprocity, and sustainability?

The conviction that humanity is smarter than nature might be our downfall, as Robert Oppenheimer presaged when he saw the first atomic bomb explode. Quoting the Bhagavad Gita he said, "Now I am become death, the destroyer of worlds." The belief that nature can be outsmarted has created the bubble in which we now find ourselves trapped. From an early age, we are indoctrinated to believe that we can manufacture nature and replace her benefits with commodities we can buy. We are told that to be happy and healthy we need only wealth and material goods. Meanwhile the things we really need to be happy and healthy—human connection, good nourishment, exercise, connection to nature—are made more difficult in our socially stratified and disconnected world.

While the roots of our divorce from the natural world may be found in Cartesian thinking and the seventeenth-century scientific revolution, they also undoubtedly brought humankind many benefits. Over the past 300 years, we have discovered the biological basis for many illnesses and developed effective treatments for the infectious causes of millions of deaths for generations. Advances like vaccines and sterile surgical techniques and birth control have minimized the risk involved in childbirth and childhood and dramatically increased our life expectancies. Technologies increasing the efficiency of food production and distribution have dramatically decreased deaths from famine.

But in the last few years, we've started to see the gains in life expectancies level off and have even seen them drop in many rich countries. It's possible that other influences on human health and wellness are overwhelming our ability to engineer biology through the tools of science and technology alone.

A new way of thinking that leverages a reciprocal relationship with the natural world rather than trying to bend, manipulate, and conquer her may be the way forward. Our healthcare system is the logical place to expect such guidance on creating healthy lives, and at one time traditional healers did concern themselves with the way community and relationships affected well-being. We now call these factors the social determinants of health, and they account for about 80 percent of our overall wellness—but they are relegated to the margins of our modern healthcare system. How did the practice of medicine come to ignore the vast majority of what we humans need to be healthy?

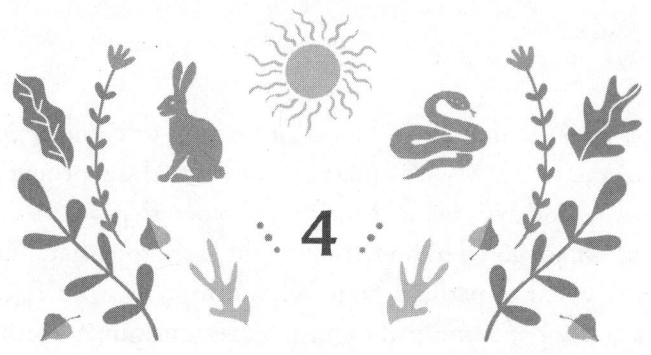

Gardens or Machines

Medicine is a social science, and politics is just
medicine practiced on a large scale.

—RUDOLPH VIRCHOW

I often feel like the victim of a bait and switch. I was sold an expensive medical education on the premise that I'd learn how to cure illness and help people stay healthy. If I had known that my chosen profession addressed only about 20 percent of what determines a person's health, that the focus of my education would be on treatments aimed mostly at the latest stages of disease, that many of those wouldn't be very effective, and finally that a large portion of the population wouldn't have access to those services, it might have given me pause before embarking on my medical career.

Thirty years ago, at The Ohio State University College of Medicine, I was taught to methodically break down the human body into its smallest components (sometimes quite literally in gross anatomy lab). In the first year I learned the name of each constituent part, down to the nerves controlling each muscle and all of the skull's foramen—the tiny holes in bone that allow blood and nerves to communicate with the rest of the body. My classmates and I learned the proper function of the organs and systems as if they were separate gears in a machine. Scant time was devoted to how they might work together. The second year was devoted to pathology, to what can go awry if a gear breaks or wears out, or if some pathogen invades and gums up the works, then we learned about the procedures and the medications we could summon to treat and cure.

The final two years were dedicated to putting it all together as apprentices in clinical settings. We were taught about hospitals and hierarchies and how to apply all we learned in books to "real life." Unfortunately, real life was messier than we'd been led to believe. Patients didn't take their medicines, they failed to follow through on our evidence-based plans, and sometimes they didn't show up at all. They behaved in ways that seemed antithetical to their own well-being. They drank, they smoke, they worked in dangerous jobs, they had risky sex, they ate junk food. Simply informing them of the error of their ways seldom made much difference.

Throughout four years of medical school, we were hyper-focused on the individual. We dissected and examined everything under those outer layers of the epidermis down to the innermost cells that make up our blood and bile. We learned almost nothing about the forces on the other side of our protective dermatological coverings, or that those forces might have more profound effects on the body's functioning than any of the biological processes we spent all our time memorizing. Much of the basic science we learned was important, but it's a small part of what determines our mental and physical wellness. I left medical school poorly prepared to understand the factors that determine 80 percent or more of my patients' health.

There's a parable told in public health circles. A physician is like a rescuer standing on the side of a river. We see a person drowning and jump in to save them, then we see another and rescue them, and then another. We are too busy pulling people out to stop and question why people are falling into the river in the first place. Much of my time in clinical practice is spent pulling people out of that river, drying them off a bit, giving them a short pep talk about how to swim, then pushing them right back into the river—to unhealthy environments, abusive relationships, stressful jobs, and poverty. On many days, it seems futile. I bring to bear all my accumulated medical knowledge to devise an airtight treatment plan, carefully adjust the doses of medication, assiduously educate my patients about their diseases and how to manage them, only to send them back to impossible environments where I know they will be hard-pressed to implement anything we just discussed.

After a few years of practice, the search for a better way brought me to public health school at Johns Hopkins University. I wanted to understand more fully the factors that caused people to get dumped into the toxic river in the first place. Now, after years of education and decades of practice, I can articulately pontificate and cite evidence about those factors, the social determinants of health. In my day-to-day clinical practice though, there is still very little I can do to help my individual patients navigate and "treat" those root causes.

Building Trust

By all medical reasoning and probability, Antonia has far outlived her life expectancy. For years she has struggled with sleep apnea, emphysema, and diabetes. She comes to only about half her appointments with me. She does not always answer her phone and her voicemail is generally full, or her phone is temporarily "out of service." When my nursing staff does reach her to remind her of an appointment or refill a medication, she is rude to them more often than not. She takes her medication and uses her oxygen only sporadically, so her diabetes is usually far out of control. When she does manage a visit, her percent of blood oxygen saturation is often down in the 80s—not good. She refuses to use a CPAP machine to help her breathe at night because she lives in a small home with many family members and she doesn't want to bother them with the noise. Sometimes her various ailments get bad enough to send her to the hospital for a few nights, but she always bounces back.

I have to believe that one of the reasons that Antonia continues to survive, despite all odds, is the power of healing relationships in her life, with her family and with me. She often tells me that I "saved her life," although clinically I can't justify that statement. Sure, I have encouraged her to take her insulin more regularly, to go for more walks, and even marginally improve her diet, and maybe those things have nudged her vital signs and laboratory tests a little more in the positive direction, but she still astounds me every time I see her. When she does come into the clinic or when we talk on the phone, we mostly discuss her life and her family. I don't spend time cajoling her to get a mammogram because after eight years of trying, I know it's futile. We almost always start and end our clinic visits with a big hug. Antonia trusts me and she knows that I deeply care for her, so when I tell her something is critically important, like checking her blood sugars or using her oxygen, she listens. And I listen to her too, so when she tells me she doesn't want any screening exams for cancers because she'd rather not know and leave it up to God, I respect her decision and I don't push it, resisting the urge to cast so much as a disapproving glance.

Over the past twenty-five years, I think I have become a pretty good doctor. My clinical knowledge has deepened considerably, but even now I liberally look up diagnostic criteria, drug dosing, and recommended treatments on one of my many medical apps. Most of the improvements in my healing skills have not come from memorizing more facts but from honing my medical intuition. We doctors don't talk about intuition in medicine very much, and when we do, it's mostly to disparage its importance. Our teachers tell us that intuition is not "evidence-based" and might lead us astray. I think that's a false dichotomy. I've learned that intuition comes from the strength of the relationships and trust I have with my patients. The combination of evidence-based clinical knowledge, years of experience, listening skills, and empathy is powerful medicine.

We are not taught in medical school how to listen to our patients, and in our current profit-driven healthcare system, there is very little time or space for relationship building. As a result, Americans' trust in their doctors and the healthcare system has eroded dramatically. In 1966, more than three-fourths of Americans had "great confidence" in medical leaders; now only 34 percent do. Only a quarter of Americans today say they have faith in the healthcare system as a whole.[1] During the coronavirus pandemic, we saw everywhere the consequences of the lack of trust in our public health institutions. The refusal to wear masks or follow stay-at-home and social-distancing directives cost many thousands of lives. Skepticism about vaccinations delayed our emergence from the crisis and cost thousands more.

Much of the distrust and dissatisfaction may be due to the unpleasant experiences many of us have had in clinics and hospitals. Even those with insurance and financial means have difficulties accessing compassionate care, or they find themselves with huge bills for hidden costs. National Public Radio and Kaiser Health News have a popular series about "surprising medical bills." There is no problem finding stories for the program. Listeners have sent accounts of six stitches that cost over $6,000, a $54,000 COVID test, and a NICU stay that cost an insured family over $500,000 (the hospital graciously offered to let them pay it off in monthly installments of $45,843 over a year).[2] Even with these exorbitant costs, the demand for healthcare far outstrips the supply, and long waits for appointments are becoming the norm.

Once we are finally able to get in to see the doctor, many of us leave the exam room feeling misunderstood, dismissed, unheard and even belittled. Over the years, several studies have measured the amount of time that doctors allow patients to speak before interrupting, with the average from a 2018 study clocking in at eleven seconds.[3] During the short fifteen or twenty minutes generally allocated for a visit, physicians feel we must immediately take control and steer the conversation to the things we have been taught are most important. There is no space or time for patients to tell us about their family and personal relationships, about their home or work lives, about their joys and sorrows, or anything else that doesn't relate directly to some physical symptom or biological process. We are taught to redirect patients and focus on the subjects about which we are knowledgeable. We demand patients conform to our medical paradigm, rather than the other way around. We are instructed to tell the patient to limit themselves to just one or two "problems," but how is the patient to know which is more important? The nagging back pain, or the bloating, or the small insignificant mole on their arm that might just be a fatal melanoma? Few of us have learned much about the healing power of relationships, and many doctors eschew such subjects as unimportant to their work. After all, how could these "psychosocial" elements possibly be relevant to a neurosurgeon or emergency medicine doctor? But trust building and deep listening are useful in almost any situation.

Several years ago, I was on a long-haul flight from Seattle to Amsterdam. Shortly after takeoff the familiar call came: "Is there a doctor on the flight?" I got up and was joined by an EMT and internal medicine physician. An older Chinese woman in the first row had developed shortness of breath and chest pain. The EMT and the internal medicine doctor immediately wanted to start an IV and give her oxygen and nitroglycerin. After seeing that her vital signs were stable, I sat down quietly next to her and asked about her health. She had no medical problems and saw her doctor regularly. Then I asked her why she thought she was experiencing this distress. Through the scant English she knew, she explained that it was always her responsibility to order the flowers for Sunday morning church service, and she had forgotten to tell anyone that she was traveling and wouldn't be able to do it. She felt terribly anxious and guilty at having let her congregation down. When I told her that I'd be happy to text someone for her as soon as we were able, she calmed down and felt better immediately. The EMT, however, still insisted on starting an IV.

It's hard to quantify the power of trust in the healing relationship; it can't be easily measured by a randomized controlled trial, that holy grail of Western medical knowledge. In fact, the randomized controlled trial is only one "way of knowing" and certainly not the best one in all situations.[4] There are other, equally valid empirical methods that are just as "scientific."[5]

The placebo effect is one phenomenon difficult to explain solely through randomized controlled trials. Latin for "I shall please," placebos are most commonly thought of as a sugar pill with no biological effect, but in reality they can be anything, like a ceremony or ritual. Placebo surgeries, which involve just making a random incision in the skin, have been shown to improve conditions like chronic pain. Although there are a variety of mechanisms that seem to be involved in the placebo effect, they may be rooted in patient's expectations. We are more likely to believe in a treatment if we trust the person administering it. Placebos work not so much because of the individual's faith in the placebo itself, but more because of trust or belief in the person or situation surrounding the placebo. The power is magnified in the context of a compassionate healing relationship.[6]

Healing Before There Was Healthcare

Long before what we call our "healthcare system" or "medicine" existed, there were healers. Since the dawn of human history, medicine people have had an honored place in human societies. Medicine may truly be the oldest profession. In almost all parts of the world, traditional healers still do their work, sometimes alongside but mostly at odds with Western medicine.

In the days before "modern" medicine, Indigenous healers, midwives, and shamans had few tools to use beyond their relationship with their patients, a shared cultural history, and knowledge of the natural world that surrounded them. Exposure to this way of healing has been all but stamped out of Western medical education, trampled by an infatuation with reductionist biological processes, technology, and pharmaceuticals. Dr. Bernard Lown, the inventor of the cardiac defibrillator, writes in *The Lost Art of Healing* that "practicing the art of medicine requires not only expert knowledge of disease but an appreciation of the intimate details of a patient's emotional life. . . .

The need for complex involvement with patients is never alluded to in medical texts or mentioned during medical training."

During my time in Mozambique helping scale up HIV treatment in government-run clinics, I quickly learned that most Mozambicans with HIV hedged their bets. They would avail themselves of the medicines we offered, but they also frequented traditional healers, known as curandeiras, and faith healers, called profetas. These individuals were respected members of the local community and had likely known the patient and their extended family since birth. The "alternative" healers used their cultural and spiritual ties with the communities, along with personal relationships and knowledge of local medicinal plants, to treat all manner of ailments of heart, mind, body, and soul. The combination of all three healing modalities was the most effective integrated response to HIV and AIDS.

Just a few hundred years ago, allopathic Western medicine—the dominant brand of medicine practiced in the US today—was just one of many healing traditions available in Europe and the Americas, and it wasn't considered superior. Throughout the eighteenth and nineteenth centuries there were no systemic scientific methods or randomized controlled trials applied to allopathic cures. One could make the case that many traditional healers, with centuries of empirical observation passed down through generations, had a stronger scientific basis for their practice. A study done in the early 1900s supported this idea and showed that traditionally trained and experienced midwives had better outcomes for their patients than the university-trained obstetricians of the time.[7]

Traditional healers were among the first practitioners of empiric methods. They observed the cause and effects of their treatments and passed that knowledge on to younger practitioners. The effectiveness of medicines discovered this way has been borne out time and again by modern scientific study. To name just a few, we owe aspirin, digoxin, morphine, some malaria medications, statins, and many anti-cancer drugs to the original research of traditional healers. About 11 percent of the medications on the WHO list of essential medicines are derived from natural sources, almost all originally discovered by Indigenous peoples. Even the first vaccines were based on the scientific studies of Asian and North African practitioners in the sixteenth century or earlier. Through careful observation, they discovered that inoculation with cowpox would prevent patients from developing the more fatal smallpox disease. These healthcare providers were the first to come up with the innovation of intentionally infecting their patients with a less pathogenic version of an illness to protect them against the lethal version, a practice we now call immunization, and one that has saved millions of lives.[8]

Instead of building on and integrating this rich history of "folk" healing knowledge passed down for generations, European and American allopathic doctors felt threatened by it. They were almost all university-educated white men from elite families, in contrast to the mostly poorer men and women and people of color who practiced so-called natural or traditional medicine passed on from ancestors. In Europe, the need to crush alternative forms of healing led directly to the persecution and genocide of mostly women healers and midwives during the witch hunts of the Middle Ages. In the United States, the elite banded together to fund university-based medical schools at places like Johns Hopkins and Harvard, while at the same time creating licensing laws to outlaw alternative forms of medicine. The sole path to becoming a doctor and legally practicing medicine had to start with a degree from a state-sanctioned university. Anyone else delivering a baby or offering a remedy to a sick child would run the risk of prosecution. In this way, the medical profession was purged of nearly everyone except white men for most of the twentieth century.

The origins of Western medicine may explain why traditional forms of healing were disparaged and ignored. One of medicine's main goals throughout the eighteenth and nineteenth centuries was to help European men stay healthy as they carried out the imperial project. Fixing soldiers so that they could return to battle and curing infectious diseases like malaria were integral to successful colonization. To this day we still use metaphors of war to describe Western medical treatments. We "do battle" against cancer, and those who are cured are called "survivors."

Healers in the East took another path. Both Ayurvedic and Chinese medicine emphasize a balance between the elements in our bodies, the same elements found in nature. In Ayurveda these are ether, air, fire, water, and earth; in Chinese medicine they are wood, fire, metal, earth, water. Both Eastern healing traditions encompass treatments, like teas or pills, that are similar to Western remedies, but also are more likely to include recommendations about diet, exercise, and other kinds of behaviors. Both traditions center the importance of the mind–body connection and the patient's environment. These medical systems and many Indigenous healing traditions consider their subject's whole ecosystem and treat them much as a gardener would approach an ailing plant, asking what elements are missing or overly abundant in the environment that might be causing dysfunction. While Western medicine treats illness as an adversary to be defeated, these other modalities attempt to include outside contexts and bring equipoise to the entire system.

Machines or Gardens?

Four hundred years ago, Descartes decreed that our bodies were nothing like gardens or nature; they were more like machines, divorced from the higher essence of the mind. If we could merely observe their mechanical function, we'd unlock the secrets to healing the body and curing our ailments. He wrote: "So also the human body may be considered as a machine, so built and composed of bones, nerves, muscles, veins, blood and skin that even if there were no mind in it, it would not cease to move in all the ways it does at present when it is not moved under the direction of the will."[9]

The idea that our bodies are machines gave a framework to many valuable early discoveries in modern medicine. The germ theory in the late 1800s added another metaphor to our thinking about the body and health, that of a battlefield where we waged war against microscopic foes. These two metaphorical frames—a machine to be fixed, a war to be waged—are the twin lenses through which Western medicine has viewed the human body for the past 400 years.

During the twentieth century, between fighting and fixing, medicine addressed many scourges that caused early demises in previous centuries. Childbirth-related deaths plummeted when physicians started to employ antiseptic technique making cesarean sections safer. High infant mortality rates dropped with the introduction of antibiotics and vaccines. More-effective surgery saved many lives that would have succumbed to traumatic accidents. Remarkable advances in medicine and public health led to huge leaps in average life expectancy in the century between 1900 and 2000, from under fifty to almost seventy-five years old. Having beaten back the acute, mostly infectious diseases, we now have only chronic ailments, like cancer, diabetes, and heart disease, to vanquish. Unfortunately, they don't fit simply into machine thinking. They all have in common major environmental causal factors and can be seen as diseases with their roots in unhealthy ecosystems.

New research into subjects as varied the microbiome and immunology is beginning to shed light on another way of thinking. What if a better metaphor for our body was to view it as a garden, dependent on and in constant communication with the environment around us? For the plants in a garden to be healthy, they need adequate sun, water, and fertile soil—and they need to be protected from toxins and poisons. If we thought of the body as a garden, we might consider that cures could be found as frequently from nurturing and building resilience as from fixing what's broken or waging war against unseen enemies.

The "garden" way of thinking is slowly infiltrating medical research as new discoveries are made about the critical role a healthy microbiome plays in our well-being, or as innovative immunotherapy treatments aimed at boosting our own natural defenses are developed for cancer. Careful observers of our organism's biological systems are realizing that they are not like machines at all, but in fact complex ecosystems encompassing connections with vast numbers of other living beings both inside and outside the body. The idea of using our own immune systems to control cancer is similar to integrated pest management methods of sustainable agriculture. Rather than doing battle with a destructive enemy (whether cancer or invasive insect) by dousing it with an indiscriminate poison (chemotherapy or pesticides), natural systems themselves are bolstered to bring about a change in the environment that make conditions less favorable for the offending agent. In the case of immunological therapies for cancer, this might mean treating with specially targeted antibodies to help the immune system control or eliminate malignant tumors. This way of managing an illness echoes the approach of other modalities of medicine, like Ayurveda, or even the approach Indigenous peoples of the Americas took to managing their natural environment. The focus is on making conditions favorable for the "good" organisms and fostering an ecosystem conducive to human wellness.

For now, most of these new innovations in Western medicine are confined to different ways of considering the internal workings of our body. When it comes to understanding and addressing the ways forces outside our body might affect our health, our healthcare system is still woefully neglectful.

Health Disparities and Racism

Everything about the Western healthcare system—from pre and post-graduate training, to research, to ways of categorizing illness—emphasizes the importance of genetics and biology over environment or social factors. We need only look at the ways institutional racism can produce illness and health disparities to see how inadequate our dominant medical model is in addressing pernicious and pervasive problems rooted in our social environment.

To illustrate how racism affects health, Dr. Camara Jones, a family physician, epidemiologist, and leading public health intellectual, has invented a modern-day parable called The Gardener's Tale. The story is about a gardener with two flower boxes; one has fertile rich soil, and the other has depleted sandy soil. The gardener likes red flowers better, so she puts some red flower seeds into the good soil and pink flower seeds into the poor soil. After a while, the flowers come up, and every seed in the red flower box has sprouted into beautiful tall lush blooms. The pink flowers meanwhile have mostly died except for a few scrawny-looking stalks. The gardener harvests the seeds from the pink and the red flowers and continues to replant them into the same boxes year after year. Finally, ten years later, the gardener observes the two flower boxes and thinks to herself that she has always believed that red flowers are stronger and more beautiful, and now her own experience has shown her that she was right.

In one version of the parable, physicians play the role of the gardeners. Over and over our profession has considered the poorer health of our Black, Indigenous, and other patients of color and assumed that individual biological or behavioral factors must be leading to the disparities we see. Since our medical education is almost exclusively focused on genetic or biological causes of disease, that's where most physicians look first—hammer, meet nail. One of many examples of how this plays out comes from my own medical education. Twenty-five years ago, I learned that beta blockers, a class of medications used to treat high blood pressure, don't work as well on Black people. This point was made over and over and even made it into exam questions. The erroneous conclusion was based on small, flawed studies and has since been debunked, but old ingrained beliefs die hard. Newer review articles continue to emphasize biological differences in physiology and response to blood pressures medications among different races, even though there is scant evidence supporting this hypothesis. Specific guidelines for treating Black patients with hypertension have even been codified in the recent recommendations from the NIH's Joint National Committee on Prevention, Detection, Evaluation, and Treatment of High Blood Pressure, suggesting a narrower range of medications appropriate for these groups.[10]

The consequences of these seemingly subtle errors in our science are vast. Doctors who receive this training and follow the accepted treatment guidelines might be reluctant to use all the medications at their disposal to lower blood pressure in Black patients. As a result, blood pressures in Black patients might not be controlled as effectively, leading to other health disparities in the rates of diseases, like heart attacks and strokes, that are related to poorly controlled blood pressure. In fact, a study published in 2022 found exactly this outcome.[11] In the end, just like the Dr. Camara Jones's gardener, physicians are likely to interpret their greater challenges in treating hypertension among Black patients as just another piece of evidence reinforcing beliefs in genetic and physiological differences among patients of different races.

The misconception that race has a biological basis has a long and ignominious history with roots in attempts to justify colonization, slavery, genocide and other forms of oppression of darker-skinned peoples. When a dangerous notion like this one takes hold, it's difficult to eradicate. In my thirty-year career as a physician, not only was I never explicitly taught that racial categories are entirely human-made, but the fallacy that race is biologically determined was reinforced over and over in subtle and overt ways.

Even today, when a student presents a patient to a teaching physician, the customary way to start is listing age, race, and gender, as in "This is a thirty-three-year-old Black male," as if these are the most important identifiers. It is still rare in medical education to find explicit teaching that race is not a biological but a wholly social construct, or that no biological or genetic test can tell who is "Black." As a result, many in healthcare don't realize there has never been any evidence of biological differences between races, and therefore fail to recognize the enormous role that environment and racism have on health.

Students attending medical school today continue to make flawed assumptions that are colored by racial bias because these long-held beliefs are seldom directly challenged. A study in 2016 gave medical students two case examples, about a white patient and a Black patient in pain. The students were then asked a series of questions about the two patients. About 50 percent of medical students believed falsely that Black patients have a higher tolerance for pain because of differences in anatomy or biology, like the erroneous belief held by many in the study that Black patients have "thicker skin."[12]

While I was taught many things in medical school about race and disease that have turned out not to be true, I was never taught the one glaring fact that is true: study after study shows that the effect of race on health is mediated through the stress and the experience of racism, not biology. Dr. Camara Jones is right—our health does not so much depend on what color flower we are, but what kind of garden we are living in.

How Much Have Things Changed?

Nonwhite races are not the only groups modern medicine marginalizes. There is a clear idea of the "normal" implied and taught in medical schools—all else is considered "deviation." My own medical education was dominated by white male professors, and even the class was about 90 percent white. The general cutthroat environment and the sheer volume of work is designed to keep students a bit off-kilter and to discourage any kind of questioning of received teachings. Coming into med school, I was a like a deer in the headlights as a first-generation college kid (let alone med school). Still, I was curious about the small group of Black students and how they seemed to form their own tight-knit cohort. There were clear examples of sexism and racism, but the ones I noticed most were the those that affected me—like the time a pathology professor stood in front of a huge lecture hall with an enormous screen and showed our class of 250 students a picture of a vagina with a large tumor protruding from it while he joked that it looked like a penis going the wrong way. Some in the class snickered. I felt traumatized and wondered how the person who was pictured would feel if they knew how their image was being used. Or if they even knew that it existed.

I didn't know then that what we were learning about the supposed difference in how men and women, or different races, responded to medicines was based on scant and often-flawed studies. Or that almost all clinical research was conducted on white men of average build from Western European ancestry. We lapped up what was told to us as gospel. It was necessary for succeeding; we had to regurgitate what we were told to get honors in the rotation or pass the board exam. We learned almost nothing about how discrimination or other social factors affect health, or that people from different backgrounds or cultures might respond differently to our interventions.

Medical education has shifted somewhat, now there are LGBTQ clinics, doctors who specialize in trans care, more BIPOC and women faculty, but still the care of these populations (read: any who are not heterosexual white cis male) is considered something outside the mainstream. Department chairs and senior professors are still at least 70 percent white and male. Recently there has even been backlash against making the practice of medicine more inclusive. In February 2024, a group of dermatologists proposed to their professional association that their diversity, equity, and inclusion (DEI) programs be "sun-setted," claiming they were too divisive and created a dichotomy of "oppressor" and "oppressed." The initiative was attempting to increase the diversity in what is an overwhelmingly white specialty, as well as ensure that students and residents are taught what skin lesions look like on black or brown skin. Most dermatology textbooks and guides include only white-skinned patients, leading to a much higher frequency of misdiagnosis of skin lesions in people of color, likely contributing to worse skin cancer outcomes for those with darker skin.[13]

Where Are We Headed?

In the past thirty years, the awareness of social and environmental factors that influence health has steadily grown. Although one can now find courses in the social determinants of health and health disparities at most medical schools, they remain at the margins and often frustrate students and teachers alike. What good is it to teach about a factor that determines as much as 80 percent of our patients' health if we have few ways to address it in our healthcare system? Even as evidence mounts about the effects of the environment on our health, the field of medicine has been slow to find ways to incorporate new findings into different systems of care. In fact, it seems medicine is headed in an exact opposite, and even more reductionist, direction.

Despite what the science tells us, the newest and most lucrative trends in medicine focus ever more narrowly on the individual in hot new fields like precision and functional medicine. For those who can afford it, they promise designer cures, specifically tailored to one's unique biology and genetics. Often, what's on offer aren't even treatments for specific diseases but instead ways to "optimize" health, like diets based on genetic testing or microbiome surveys. These high-end doctors, accessible only to a wealthy few, offer of a slew of expensive laboratory and diagnostic tests not yet proven and mostly not covered by insurance.

Concierge practitioners are paid handsomely to spend hours lavishing individual attention on each patient. If those of us in "regular" medicine had this luxury, I think we'd also be able to practice better medicine even without the pricey tests. For the vast majority of us unable to afford boutique doctors, our healthcare system fails us by focusing on silver-bullet technological fixes to late-stage chronic problems while ignoring the root causes of our ailments.

The fields of functional and precision medicine are the latest evolution in a long history of mechanistic and narrow-minded clinical thinking. They are both based on the premise that unlocking the secrets of our genome will finally reveal the inner workings of our machine body and allow us to fix any ailment. Despite the fact the Human Genome Project finished mapping our DNA twenty years ago, fewer than expected medical advances have emerged, mostly focused on better cancer treatments. Ongoing research might provide cures for an array of genetic diseases, but likely won't much affect the diseases that account for the most common causes of morbidity and mortality, those pernicious chronic illnesses like heart disease and diabetes.

One reason deciphering our genetic code seems to have failed so far to yield promised benefits may have to do with new information about how the genome interacts with our environment. Previous thinking was that our DNA was like a blueprint for a fully functional human being. If we figured out the blueprint and found the "mistakes" that created disease, we could just overwrite the flawed section. A better analogy is that the genome is more like a database of blueprints, many of which may never be used to make anything. The key to what determines which blueprints are used—the expression of genes, and the ways certain genes are turned on or off—likely has much more to do with how and why some people develop illnesses and others do not. The field of epigenetics is just starting to explore the myriad ways our environment influences our genes, from histories of trauma that can affect mental health generations later, to why cancers are more common in some areas, to why some people develop diabetes or heart disease while their genetically similar siblings do not. Even applied to the understanding of our own genome, seeing our bodies as ecosystems or gardens is more accurate and helpful than the outdated trope of the body as a machine.

Changing the Frame

Shifting the frame seems like a daunting task. Over one million physicians and four million nurses currently practicing in the United States have been trained to think about patients in a mechanistic and individualized way. Our healthcare system depends on financial reimbursements tied mostly to tests or procedures, not on time spent getting to know patients, their families, and their communities. Although recent billing changes allow consideration for how healthy patients are or the length of primary care visits, we still have a profit-based healthcare system that demands laser focus on what is considered a "billable service."

Many others before me have called for critically examining our medical school, pre-med, and other health science curricula, and indeed medical education has evolved in the thirty years since I was a student, but the basic structure remains in most places—two years of mostly memorization of the fundamentals of the human body and its pathologies, followed by two years of clinical experience, mainly in hospitals where the sickest patients reside and are cared for by specialists. Almost all the teaching is still focused on individual factors—biology or behavior—and how they produce illness. Very little time is devoted to learning what might confer wellness and resiliency, or how a patient's living conditions and relationships affect their overall health. I have forgotten the names of all those tiny holes in the base of the skull, and since I am not a neurosurgeon, at no point have my patients suffered because I can no longer locate the foramen spinosum on an anatomy model. They have been hurt, however, by doctors who assume that their afflictions are caused by biology or personal failings rather than toxic environments. What if some of that specialized instruction was moved to the residencies of specialists who need that knowledge, and medical school focused more on the information every future doctor needs?

All healthcare providers need to know how to listen, have empathy, and build trust in our communications with patients. This subject is virtually ignored in medical education. Doctors learn instead how to take a "medical history," which consists largely of a checklist of information to be ticked off. If an aspect of a patient's story doesn't fit into the checklist, the implicit conclusion is that it's not important. All health professional students need to learn very early and unequivocally about the social determinants of health and that racial health disparities are caused by institutional racism and not biological difference. Many of us bring years of conditioned assumptions about race and racism to medical school that lead us to different conclusions. Medical education must directly confront, challenge, and overcome those erroneous ideas.

The healthcare delivery system must also be revamped. First and foremost, we must demand a healthcare system that is affordable and accessible to all. Maya Angelou famously said, "No one of us can be free until everybody is free." If our individual health depends on the health of our communities, then it is also true that no one can be truly healthy unless we are all healthy, or at least have access to the same conditions and requirements for our well-being.

The very conception of healthcare and the doctor's visit should be dramatically changed. Even if doctors got better training on social and environmental influences on health, we can't do it all alone. Having more time to build relationships with patients is just the first step. What if the healthcare system was built on integrated teams of different experts in mental health, primary care, social work, nutrition, public health, and other fields? How could all healthcare workers come together to transform the health and wellness of individuals and communities? What can be learned from centuries of traditional and Indigenous medicine? Our bodies and minds are not partitioned off into discrete silos, so neither should be our healthcare system.

Over fifty years ago, during the height of the civil rights movement, pioneering physicians and social medicine activists H. Jack Geiger, John Hatch, and Count Gibson had a vision of exactly what this different model of healthcare could accomplish. They imported the idea of community-based, multidisciplinary healthcare from a clinic in the South African township of Pholela, where Geiger, then a professor at Tufts University, had worked in 1957 as a medical student. Using this model, they launched what became known as the community health center movement.[14] In Judy Schader Rogers's powerful 1970 documentary *Out in the Rural*, Geiger had this to say about the vision for the first such center in Mound Bayou, Mississippi, which opened in 1967:

> *What kind of a place are we? I think we're a place that has as its primary thesis that the determinants of health are in the social order, not in health care. I've never seen any use in . . . the idea that you stand around in whatever circumstances, laying hands on people in the traditional medical way—waiting until they're sick, curing them—and then sending them back unchanged into an environment that overwhelmingly determines that they're going to get sick.[15]*

He too was tired of pushing people back into the toxic river. The revolutionary idea was that these health centers—deeply embedded in the community—would not just cure diseases but also address the root causes of illness, from poor access to healthy foods to lack of education, housing, and employment. After securing grants from Tufts and President Lyndon Johnson's Office of Economic Opportunity, Geiger, Hatch, and Gibson did more than just build a clinic in an area without reliable access to healthcare: they also dug wells and established a library, farm cooperative, and office of education. When his patients were malnourished, Geiger wrote prescriptions for food to be purchased at local, Black-owned grocery stores and paid out of the pharmacy's budget. "The last time I looked in my medical textbooks," he told a federal official after the governor complained, "they said the specific therapy for malnutrition was food."[16]

The Delta Health Center in Mississippi still exists today, along with its sister pilot clinic in the Columbia Point area of Dorchester. Joining them, the community health center movement has grown into a network of over 1,300 federally supported clinics serving 28 million patients of all backgrounds and income levels—all focused on providing excellent primary care to those who need it most, regardless of their ability to pay. The federal government requires community health center boards to reflect the demographic makeup of their communities; at least half the board has to be made up of current patients.

I became a convert to the community health center movement early in my career when I was matched into the Northern New Mexico Family Medicine Residency and started seeing patients at La Familia Medical Center in Santa Fe. I saw a kind of medicine that started to make sense, where community health workers and diabetes educators and counselors and nurse practitioners and doctors worked together, all focused on everything patients needed to be healthy. I could see a patient, diagnose their early diabetes, and then call in a peer who spoke their language, understood their culture, and could spend an hour or more explaining their condition and then work with the patient to create a plan for improving their health that considered all the potential social and environmental barriers. The training I received in residency colored my entire medical career.

After fifteen years away, I returned to La Familia to serve as medical director in 2012. There, with a team of other compassionate, intelligent, and highly dedicated healthcare workers, we were able to create many innovative programs to address the social determinants of health. Two of these stand out as special examples of what's possible when healthcare is delivered with consideration of a patient's whole ecosystem. One was called CENA, which means "dinner" in Spanish but is also an acronym for Comunidad, Ejecicio, Nutrición y Acción (Community, Exercise, Nutrition and Action). Families struggling with nutrition and weight were referred by our providers to a team that included a nutritionist and a community health worker. The whole family was assessed and screened for health problems like hypertension, obesity, and early diabetes, then the family joined a community of other families in the program. There were cooking classes, group visits to the farmer's markets, and family-centered exercise excursions like group hikes. Families were also enrolled in a program that provided them with a customizable "basket" of healthy foods every week at steep discounts. The program was incredibly popular and the cooking classes filled to capacity with thirty or more attendees. Participating patients reported improving their diets and exercising more and generally feeling healthier, even after just a few months.

The second initiative came about when the clinic made a commitment to address the worsening opioid overdose epidemic, which had deep roots in our northern New Mexico communities. I was so proud of our provider group when almost all agreed to complete the training necessary to prescribe a lifesaving medicine called buprenorphine, which, like methadone, is extremely effective in treating opioid addiction and dependence. Our team, led by Mexican-trained physician Myriam Salazar, included social and housing support, referrals to counseling, and treatment for associated illnesses like hepatitis C. Myriam and her staff treated our patients like family and would call or even visit patients at home when they didn't come in for appointments.

Photographer and filmmaker Jackie Munro led a storytelling project, coaching patients on the use of high-end cameras. The resulting videos and photo-stories were so powerful that Ira Glass invited the young mothers in the program to tell their stories during a performance at Santa Fe's Lensic Theater. The program was one of the earliest integrating buprenorphine treatment seamlessly into primary care, and our results were impressive, with over 50 percent of patients still in treatment after six months.

Although community health centers are among the few places in this country where healthcare workers have the opportunity to address at least some of the root causes that determine most of our well-being, it's still not possible in most places to write prescriptions and have them honored for housing or healthy foods or adequate transportation as envisioned by Dr. Geiger, though these would cost less per month than many medications for late-stage illness that *are* covered. Even when healthcare workers create programs like those I've described, they struggle for funding and sustainability because addressing the social determinants of health is not envisioned by the current system of healthcare financing and reimbursements in the United States.

Good evidence shows that what we currently consider the practice of medicine only addresses about 20 percent of what makes us healthy. The other 80 percent is contained in the context of our lives—that mix of environment, status, community, stress, family, work, and ancestry—almost entirely ignored by our healthcare system. Focusing on just that last 20 percent is like fielding a soccer team with only a goalie. Most of those root causes are creating suffering and illness not only for humans but for other living things as well. As long as we insist on looking at disease and wellness exclusively through a biological lens, we will miss out on comprehending the importance of the ecosystems on which we depend. Western medicine has been complicit in selling us the delusion that our health is separate from the health of the earth by focusing on just a narrow sliver of what constitutes our well-being, failing to address most of what determines our health, tinkering around the edges while ignoring the major forces which undermine our quality of life. How would we look at ourselves differently if we internalized the knowledge that we are ecosystems within ecosystems rather than individual genetically determined beings? Let's start to change the frame by understanding our own bodies not as single organisms, but more accurately as communities of living things.

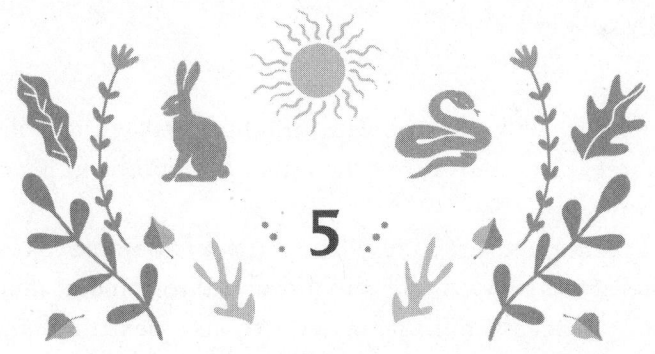

Our Bodies Are Ecosystems

[The] biggest difference between our modern human lives and the way we used to live is not the difference of housing styles and convenience. . . . It is instead the change in our web of ecological connections. We have gone from lives immersed in nature to lives in which nature appears to have disappeared."

—ROB DUNN, *THE WILD LIFE OF OUR BODIES*

"I think the yeast is causing everything."

The woman in my exam room felt sure she finally found the common thread linking all her mysterious maladies. Yeast explained her rash, her dull-colored brittle nails, thin hair, chronic fatigue, the bloating, reflux, and her depression. She was the third patient that day completely convinced that a candida overgrowth was the root of all that was afflicting her. She wondered if I could prescribe a pill or maybe a special diet.

Patient after patient tells me their story of general malaise and vague symptoms, sure their distress is related to something outside themselves. Some days it's yeast, some days it's parasites. They are partly right—their health problems might be related to a disordered microbiome, or dysbiosis. But the crux of the problem is not simply foreign invaders.

We have learned just enough about the microbiome to be dangerous. The new knowledge is shoehorned into a medical-industrial model to produce simplistic answers to complex problems. These often come in the form of individually targeted miracle cures, neatly packaged and sold in social media ads. Our microbiome is an inherent part of us. When things go awry, the culprit is usually not a single interloper but a complex imbalance of myriad organisms that evolved with us in an intricate ecosystem, intimately connected to the environment around us. My patients see themselves as isolated individuals under attack by "bad" germs rather than just one of many beings in a complex web of relationships that is more like a garden in need of tending than a fortress being sieged.

I can't blame my patients for falling victim to the black-and-white thinking promoted by alternative and conventional healthcare providers alike. Although there are many responsible cutting-edge scientists and health professionals bringing attention to the critical importance of the microbiome and developing innovative therapies, new ideas also attract a slew of opportunists looking to make a buck. They sell expensive testing kits and then prescribe personalized plans, diets, or supplements—all based on scant evidence. Judging from the people of all ages and backgrounds I see in my family medicine practice, many of us have bought what they're selling.

Most of the "cures" offered are hyper-focused on the individual and require buying something pricey—a diet, a program, a pill. But what if our external environment itself is not capable of supporting our internal ecosystem? And what about the conflicting advice? How do we know when we really might need that antibiotic, or which probiotic we should take, or which diet we should follow, or whose book we should buy? And what if none of that matters as much as our personal connections to each other, to nature, and the amount of stress or harmful substances we encounter in our lives?

Unfortunately, restoring a dysfunctional microbiome is much more complicated than knowing your gut type, taking a special pill, or eating more yogurt—it requires a new lens through which to view health and wellness. Your body itself is an ecosystem, dependent on millions of intricate relationships. Medical science understands only a tiny fraction of them. To cure our malaise, we need a whole new frame. Forging new relationships with the microorganisms that share our bodies starts with understanding how our individual quest for wellness is connected to the well-being of the whole planet, rather than an us-against-the-world battle.

It can be difficult to comprehend the depth of our dependence on the microbiome because it goes against everything we've been taught about germs and health. To see how very ingrained that thinking is, I have to take you back to my medical school years, just thirty years ago. There, we were taught a simple binary: antibiotics good/bacteria bad. I remember learning very little about growing issues of antibiotic resistance and almost nothing about the microbiome. We were taught that the bacteria in our gut were, at best, benign interlopers, and at worst, harmful or even deadly. They were germs, and in keeping with the germ theory, they were all suspect as potential pathogens. Bacteria were our foes to be vanquished. The implication was, if it were possible to live in a germ-free world, it would certainly be preferable. How wrong we were. The roots of this misapprehension go back even farther, to the origins of the very words we use to describe being unwell, like *illness*, *disease*, and *infection*.

A Poisonous Fog

Up until the late nineteenth century, in Europe the prevailing belief held by both scientists and laypeople was that all maladies had their roots in toxic air emanating from rotting food, swamps, sewage, or dirty water. The invisible poisonous fog was called "miasma," thus this theory of how diseases arise is known as the miasma theory. It was believed that if one was exposed to proverbial bad air, diseases would spontaneously generate. The thought that germs caused disease was a radical new idea supported by just a few visionary thinkers and scientists, but without any hard evidence to prove it.

In the late 1800s, Louis Pasteur turned the world of medicine and science upside down when he successfully isolated the anthrax bacillus from the blood of diseased sheep and then injected the bacteria back into healthy sheep who subsequently developed anthrax, thereby establishing that a single identifiable microorganism caused a specific disease without any help from bad air. This was the revolutionary proof needed for a groundbreaking theory.

The germ theory caught on quickly. An explosion of scientific advances followed the work of Pasteur and many others, undoubtedly saving millions of lives. This new way of seeing the world would lead to effective antibiotics for infectious disease, vaccines, and improved surgical outcomes.

Pasteur himself developed some of the first intentionally designed vaccines against anthrax and rabies. A young English surgeon, Dr. Joseph Lister, took the theory and applied it to wound infections. He developed and promulgated the first antiseptic techniques, turning surgery from a long-odds gamble to a lifesaving treatment. The new procedures, applied to difficult childbirths and cesarean sections, contributed dramatically to sharp decreases in maternal and infant mortality in the early twentieth century.

Malaria was among the first infectious diseases targeted after the germ theory gained acceptance. Fittingly, malaria gets its name from Latin for "bad air" and was long thought to come from a dangerous gas given off by swamps. Until the early twentieth century, malaria was prominent in both Europe and the United States, affecting everyone from presidents to soldiers to farmers; Washington and Lincoln both had it. By the turn of the century, the parasite's life cycle was described, and mosquitos were identified as the offending vector, transmitting the tiny microbe when they fed on human blood. The main response to malaria, cleansing our environment of offending mosquitos, successfully eradicated the disease from the United States by the late 1950s but also led to widespread use of DDT and its well-known unintended consequences.[1]

The explosion of microbial research and medical advances that followed from the germ theory profoundly impacted the health of humankind. The effect can be seen most dramatically by comparing life expectancies in the hundred years between 1850 and 1950. In 1850, a white person living in the United States lucky enough to reach age 20 could only expect to live about another 20 years on average.[2] By one estimate, average life expectancy at birth for African Americans in 1850 was only 21.4 years.[3] Fully one-fifth of white children and one-third of African American children died before their first birthday. By 1950, life expectancy at birth had soared to almost 70 years for whites and 60 for African Americans. Infant mortality rates had dropped to one in thirty (although racial disparities persist to this day).[4] The advances made possible by the germ theory explain almost all the difference.

The message encoded in these advances was clear: germs were harmful and needed to be eradicated wherever they were hiding. In the century that followed, we declared war on all microorganisms, be they virus, bacteria, fungus, parasite, or even insect. This mentality, demonstrated to be so effective in the eradication of malaria, was applied to everything that seemed unclean or offensive. Pesticides proliferated and were wantonly and indiscriminately applied without much thought regarding their safety for non-targeted beings, including humans. Antibiotics were handed out like candy to anyone with so much as a sneeze. The chemical industry seized the opportunity and capitalized on our intense fear of germs. A proliferation of corporations continues to sell us new and improved ways every year to create a chemically enhanced barrier between us and the natural germ-filled world. Today we can find antiseptic products specifically designed for every nook and cranny of our lives. Antimicrobials have found their way into our soaps, makeup, paints, and even our clothing.

The Rest of the Story

For all its accomplishments, germ theory only told half the story. Listening carefully to those who first developed the theory, one can hear the nuance in their thinking. Pasteur himself was a strong advocate for killing the harmful microbes in milk but thought that most microbes were obligate mutualists, meaning that we needed each other, man and microbe, to survive. Russian scientist Élie Metchnikoff, one of the founders of the field of immunology, was also one of the earliest longevity researchers. In his book *The Prolongation of Life: Optimistic Studies*, he proposed that aging is caused by an overgrowth of toxic bacteria and suggested that ingesting good lactobacillus bacteria could help lengthen life. To prove his theory, he drank sour milk regularly, and it seems to have worked. He died in 1916 at the age of seventy-one, beating the average life expectancy for his time by about thirty years. Metchnikoff and Pasteur's early hunches have proved true. Yes, germs cause disease, but they also are essential for our well-being. And sometimes the same germ can be in both categories, harmful in some situations, helpful in others.

Recent realizations about the importance of a germy environment to human health are as significant as the shift from the miasma theory to the germ theory in the 1800s. With the past decade's explosion of research, the picture of the microbiome has come into much richer focus since the black-and-white "bacteria bad/antibiotics good" binary I was taught in the early 1990s. We now know that for every human gene in our bodies, there are 360 microbial ones, and that the cells of microorganisms outnumber our human cells by ten to one.[5]

We've learned much from the significant investment in the Human Microbiome Project, launched in 2007, and similar sister projects in Europe, China, Canada, Ireland, South Korea, and Japan. A healthy microbiome is critical for many of our basic bodily functions, with more being discovered every day. The microbial mix in and on our bodies affects

- Digestion and how food is processed in the body

- Propensity for obesity, heart disease, cancer, dementia and other chronic diseases

- The proper functioning of the immune system

- The supply and metabolism of key vitamins and neurotransmitters

- The endocrine system and hormonal regulation

- Levels of stress

- Sleep patterns

- Variation in response to certain drugs

- Moods, general mental health, and susceptibility to depression

- The general level of inflammation in the body

The microbial ecosystem influences health from womb to the tomb. We now know that whether babies are born vaginally or by cesarean section and whether they are breastfed have profound effects on their microbiome throughout their lifespan. The development of our immune system from infancy is intimately related to our microscopic fellow travelers, and the list of illnesses and conditions linked to the microbiome is growing every day. It includes preterm labor, diabetes, inflammatory bowel disease, gum infections and cavities, autism, and schizophrenia. The organisms we go through life with are an integral part of us. They live in our nose and mouth, in our guts and genitalia, they coat our skin. They are not something outside our being, they are part of our being. Our wellness depends on a healthy array of microbes, and together we are superorganisms, or *holobionts*, a term coined to describe the dependent and necessary relationships between all symbiotic living things that make up our body.[6] Put another way, your body is actually an ecosystem and not an isolated individual organism.

These bacterial brethren have been with us all along, though we may be just discovering them. They have accompanied us throughout our evolution from hominids to humans, from hunter-gatherers to agrarians to city dwellers. Along the way, we and our microbes adapted and shifted in response to each other and the many challenges we faced from our changing environment.

Ancestral Microbiomes

My grandmother grew up in a cottage nestled among the Carnic Alps of northern Italy, a village called Forni di Sotto. Forni is at the base of a dramatic granite bowl, surrounded by mountains on three sides with a still-pristine trout stream forming the fourth boundary. Like most Italian mountain towns, the village is densely packed with boxy brick and wooden buildings huddled around a central square. Bucolic pastures dotted with household gardens, fenced to keep out woodland creatures and errant goats, form a buffer between the homes and the steep slopes.

In the early 1900s, when my grandmother was young, she and her family spent the summers in their mountain house, about a half-mile walk up the side of a mountain from their village home. They stayed on the second floor of the stone cabin while the farm animals, goats and chickens and cows, would shelter on the ground floor. She and her brothers spent their days in the forest tending livestock, gathering wild herbs, and catching fish and frogs in the river to bring home for dinner. Decades later, she still vividly recalled how the freshly skinned frogs' legs twitched in the bowl as her mother floured and fried them. They consumed cheeses, yogurt, and wines transformed magically from milk and grapes by specific local yeasts.

Food preparation was a visceral act, involving all the senses and minimal utensils. I learned from my mother and grandmother how to make pasta with bare hands—first heaping a mountain of flour, then making a crater for the eggs and working the wet and dry ingredients to perfect consistency, then finally rolling the dough to the precise thickness and filling each ravioli by hand. If we look back just a few generations, most of us would find our great-great-grandparents engaged in similar pursuits with a continual exchange of microorganisms between their bodies and the world around them. *Terroir* is the idea that unprocessed foods maintain the flavor of their place, but people and their bodies also have a kind of terroir, the influences of the place they are rooted, mixed with bits and pieces of where their ancestors came from. Just as wine takes on the flavor of the land where it's cultivated, so do we.

Not all of us are lucky enough to have imbibed wisdom directly from our grandmothers. Some have had the links to our nature-embedded past brutally severed by histories of colonization, forced migration, slavery, and genocide. We may not know or remember our ancestors' stories of how they lived, but our bodies remember in our tastes for certain foods, or the way we respond to milk or wheat, or in our propensity for illnesses like sickle-cell anemia or diabetes. They may be labeled "diseases" now, but those genetic relics once kept our great-great-grandparents alive long enough to give birth to our forebears. Our human species' adaptations to place; our ability to coexist with the specific ecosystem that was found in Mozambique in the year 213 CE, in Siberia in 2000 BCE, or Laos 500 years ago; and our facility to make common cause with some microbes and détente with others are exactly the reasons that any of us are here today.

We inherit from our ancestors a unique genetic code that developed in concert with the specific web of connections from our places of origin. Our bodies evolved in response to the microbes that surrounded them, in many cases to the symbiotic advantage of both ourselves and the creatures around us. Gary Nabhan, in his book *Food, Genes, and Culture*, observes, "Ethnic cuisine reflects the evolutionary history of a particular human population as it responded to the availability of edible plants and animals through local foraging and through trade, and to the prevailing frequencies of diseases, droughts, and plagues within each population's homeland."[7] When it's working well, our internal ecosystem is attuned to our external environment and our place in the world, including the foods, soil, and microbes that are native to that place. This relationship is in constant flux, responding to changes in diet or diseases or climate. In real ways, our microbiomes have their own heritage and ancestry that's intricately tied to our genetic origins.

Before the modern age, the biggest change in our ancestral ecosystems came when we shifted from being hunter-gathers to agriculturalists. That adjustment was gradual, happening over thousands of years. We entered the agricultural age slowly. Small cultivations of favorite plants became home gardens, subsistence plots, and then larger farms over centuries. Still, almost every ancient agricultural society held on to their traditions of hunting and gathering. Most of us are just two or three generations removed from grandparents who depended on a combination of locally foraged and cultivated foods.

As both hunter-gatherers and early agriculturalists, our ancestors lived in dirt, at one with, and literally enveloped by nature. By necessity, what they ate and were able to digest looked very different from the average meal we eat today. As humans slowly became place-rooted plant growers and livestock raisers, they became more dependent on agricultural products and less on foraged foods. Adaptation was critical, especially to digesting more milk and grains. At first, some of our microbe friends did the work for us, in the form of fermentation. Fermenting milk into yogurt and cheese, and grains into sourdough and injera, allowed bacteria to break down the lactose or amylose into sugars that could be more easily metabolized. Soon the little guys cut out the middleman and started setting up shop right in our bodies. Those of us with the ability to digest milk or grains owe a debt of gratitude to the process of biological evolution that occurred thousands of years ago in response to a changing diet and microbiome.

For the first many millennia of human evolution, shifts in the relationship with our microbiome happened slowly, including those influenced by agriculture and those caused by migrations. We didn't have the means yet to move quickly around the world, so we stayed close to places where our grandparents and great-grandparents lived and died. All significant moves took generations. All of that changed overnight in evolutionary terms, just the past 300 years or so. Since the Industrial Revolution, we've subjected our bodies to a microbial blender of influences, including rapid migrations, antibiotics, chemical insults, degradations of our soil, and dramatic changes in how our foods are grown and processed. Evolution can't keep up.

Human microbiomes aren't one-size-fits-all, they evolved genetically in response to specific external and internal environmental conditions, in symbiosis with our genetic selves. Recent studies support this idea, showing that while we all have some microbes in common, each of us has a specific microbial fingerprint related to our environment, genetics, and lifestyle; but unlike our actual fingerprints, our microbiome can undergo rapid alterations when conditions change.[8] As we try to make sense of this new idea of ourselves, the old medical metaphor of our bodies as machines to be maintained and periodically repaired starts to fall apart. In this emerging understanding of how our bodies function and how our well-being is determined, we once again see that we *are* gardens.

Your Body Is a Garden

My grandmother continued to cultivate her perfectly maintained backyard garden in Buffalo, New York, well into her eighties, using the bounty almost every day in home-cooked meals. I was raised on old family recipes from her region and my grandfather's—dishes like risotto, ravioli, involtini, and passatelli. When I try to replicate those dishes in my own home, they don't taste the same as I remember from my childhood. And Grandma probably lamented that her homegrown tomatoes were less tasty than the ones she recalled from her upbringing in an Alpine village.

When my grandmother moved from northern Italy to Buffalo, she had to learn how to grow different varieties of familiar vegetables. Her handwritten notes on a 1940s garden guide reveal efforts to adapt to her new environment. The smudged and worn pamphlet from Joseph Harris Co. Seed Growers of Rochester, New York, contains marginalia highlighting varieties that seem most like her memories of home, but not exactly matching. Gardens are specific to place. Certain flora will only grow in specific climates, or at certain altitudes. Even when we can grow the same varieties in disparate places, forcing our will on the environment rather than adapting to it, the tomato grown in my Santa Fe garden at 7,000 feet will taste different from the same kind grown near the shores of Lake Erie.

In addition to plants whose needs match the conditions of a specific place, gardens require fertile soil, enough sun, and plenty of water to flourish. They are exquisitely sensitive to pests and poisons, especially when stressed by drought or degraded soil. Just like gardens, our microbiome faces many threats, which have become more numerous since our civilization became industrialized and divorced from the natural environments where we and our microbes evolved together. As we unthinkingly follow the imperative of a one-sided germ theory, that we should kill all the bugs, we also poison ourselves and our world with pesticides, antibiotics, and other indiscriminate killers.

The Case for Diversity

When we wipe out all the diversity in a natural environment, harmful invasive species are more likely to find a stronghold. Take, for example, my own mortal battle against bindweed. When I moved into my house, the meadow and orchard had not been well tended for many years. There were patches of biodiversity, with native and naturalized plants like lupine, primrose, geranium, penstemon, plantain, mallow, milkweed, cota, and asters; but there were also swaths of disturbed bare dirt, overgrown raised beds, and a spotty struggling lawn. In those places where the native flora had been swept away, the invasive species found purchase, and none is more tenacious than bindweed.

Convolvulus arvensis, field bindweed, is a fast-growing morning glory vine sporting small white flowers. It first found its way to the Americas in the early 1700s, mixed with grain crop seeds imported from Europe, and easily took hold in poor soils or where other plants had been cleared. Once it finds a niche, it grows deep, widely networked roots. I often muse that the secret to longevity and rejuvenation is surely to be found in the bindweed root because no matter how many times I cut it down or dig it out, the impossible-to-kill plant will respond by growing a full-fledged vine right back from the tiniest nub left behind. When left unchecked, the dense mats of vines, leaves, and flowers choke out all other native plants or crops, greedily sucking the available nutrients from the soil and starving grasses and forbs that challenge it.

As I was contemplating how to eliminate the unwelcome bindweed mats at my home, I noticed that the relentless vine was absent from less disrupted areas. Where soil and seed and sun and rain had found their balance, local flora flourished. In my own long war against bindweed, I use several tactics. The most successful is elimination of the offending plant with careful hand-weeding and then encouraging reseeding and regrowth of native plants. After pulling up all the vine I can, I add an array of local grass and clover seeds to the now-denuded spots of lawn, rather than use one monocrop. I reseed the barren areas in the orchard with coreopsis, blue flax, and coneflower, helping them along by adding nutrients to the soil from my compost pile on a regular basis. In areas where native plants resurge, bindweed is soon diminished. Some native plants have reseeded on their own now, and not all may be completely to my liking. Many don't have pretty flowers, and a few have ingenious mechanisms of their own to propagate their species, like seeds enclosed in prickly burrs, which I spend hours detangling from my dogs' hair. I try to foster an attitude of coexistence and tolerate these less attractive plants as much as I can because they might have an essential function in the ecosystem unbeknownst to me.

In our own bodies, many microbes function like my bindweed nemesis. My patients might fear yeast or parasites, but a more dangerous foe is *Clostridiodies difficile*, commonly known as *C. diff*. Among the 500–1,000 different bacterial species in our guts at any given time, a few of the dreaded *Clostridiodies difficile* lurk in many of us, but it is usually kept in check by a vast population of other bugs. Like any invasive species, *C. diff* can take advantage and proliferate when the gut microbes are disturbed by illness, or most commonly by antibiotics. Antibiotics may work on their intended target, but they are also indiscriminate, taking out not only the cause of an infection but many of the "good" bacteria our digestive systems need to function well. Just like bindweed, *C. diff* capitalizes on barren, disturbed environments and lack of competition and quickly overwhelms. *C. diff* infections are serious, especially in the elderly or those with debilitated immune systems. At best they cause persistent diarrhea and fever; at worst, dehydration and death.

The traditional first-line treatment for an overgrowth of *C. diff* is another course of antibiotics, one specifically targeted to kill it. The approach is akin to using pesticides or herbicides on my garden, and the effect is the same. Of course much of the *C. diff* is killed, but other flora are also destroyed, and again the "land" (our digestive tract) is left bereft of its native inhabitants. What happens next depends on what grows first in the denuded space. If native flora come back quickly and strongly, they can win the day. If not, the more tenacious *C. diff* (or bindweed) will take over again. For this reason, *C. diff* often recurs in people who are unlucky enough to get infected once. Just like my bindweed, when it finds a hospitable environment, it doesn't give up easily. In recent years, aggressive strains of *C. diff* have become more common, sometimes striking even healthy young people who have not taken antibiotics. This is likely due to evolutionary pressure on the bacteria, with widespread use of antibiotics favoring more pernicious and resilient strains.

Newer treatments against *C. diff* take a more ecological approach, especially for those with recurrent illness. Antibiotics are still considered the first line, but after the slate has been wiped clean and the numbers of offending bacteria diminished, the gut is then "reseeded" and native flora are reintroduced, just as in my garden. The two reseeding methods used in medicine are probiotics, in pill form or via certain foods containing helpful bacteria and yeasts; or fecal transplants from those with healthy, well-functioning gut microbes. Although still an experimental cure, fecal transplants have a 90 percent success rate in eradicating *C. diff*.

Recently, a natural microbe storehouse has been discovered within the human body that can reseed the gut with good microbes and aid recovery after illness. It's been hiding in plain sight the whole time. Long thought to be a useless appendage dangling in the junction between the small and large intestine, the appendix seems have a critical function to perform after our gut gets overwhelmed with illness-causing viruses or bacteria. It serves a reservoir for the essential microbes necessary for critical functions of our body. When they get wiped out of the gut by a toxic invader, the appendix is a kind of seed bank and can regrow the flora your body needs to be healthy. The healthy gut biome maintained by the appendix might even be protective against colon cancer, as people who undergo appendectomies have higher risk for cancers of the digestive tract.[9]

Recharging the Microbiome, Exercising the Immune System

Not only is the balance of bacteria inside our bodies affected by what we ingest, our choice of diet or drugs, and the "anti-" or "pro-" biotics we might take, but our own internal ecosystem of thousands of organisms in our gut, on our skin, and in our mouths and noses is also in constant communication with the larger ecosystem outside our bodies.

Gardening, camping, even hiking in the forest affects our symbiotic balance. Those of us who get our hands dirty in the backyard or frequently eat homegrown or farmers market produce are constantly recharging our ecosystems with microbes from the environment. There are hundreds of beneficial microbes on a few leaves of lettuce or spinach from your garden. One common bacterium found in soil, *Mycobacterium vaccae*, has been linked to strengthening immune response to tuberculosis, decreasing stress levels, and even combating depression. New research is showing that exposure to the bacteria might help treat asthma, leprosy, and eczema as well.[10] Our body can glean these positive effects without even touching the soil; just by breathing in a natural environment, we inhale the germs through our nose.

Human beings are designed to live in the microbe-laden world. "Good" bacteria flourish when they have all the conditions they need to thrive, and they nurture and support their human hosts as well. Exposure to the "bad" bacteria is also important at a young age, when our immune systems are developing. The newly described "hygiene hypothesis" posits that living in an environment that is too sterile can have dire consequences for our health. Our immune response is like a muscle that can get stronger and more experienced at figuring out what is friend and foe when it is challenged. Researchers have studied mice raised in specially designed germ-free environments and found they are more susceptible to autoimmune diseases like ulcerative colitis and asthma compared to their germ-surrounded cousins. Infancy through childhood seems to be a particularly critical stage. If the immune system doesn't develop properly then, it's difficult if not impossible to go back and "reset" it.

If we are to take heed of what the research about how to cultivate a healthy microbiome is telling us, most of us will need to get over our aversions to "dirt" and "germs." Unfortunately, much of Western society reinforces the detrimental message that it's healthier to wall ourselves off from the natural world and the critters living there. Most of us now live in urban environments where we encounter few patches of wild plants or soil. In many poor neighborhoods, the dirt itself is toxic, holding on to lead and heavy metals from years of pollution. We have been infected with years of conditioning from the one-sided lessons of the germ theory that all bugs are bad bugs. Marketers are only too happy to capitalize on our aspirations for a germ-free life. A quick google for "antimicrobial" products brings up clothes, furniture, floor mats, sheets, towels, and even an "EnviroHygiene Orb" for $150 that emits a germ-killing UV light. To regain the intimate connection with nature so critical for our health, we will have to decondition ourselves from fears of dirt and aversion to the natural world. We will need to embrace our wildness and rewild our own bodies.

Rewilding Our Bodies

When spring comes to my valley, I eagerly await the day the ground is thawed enough so I can work the earth with my hands. I often wish I could give my grandmother a tour of my vegetable garden and orchard and wonder what wisdom she might pass on to me about how to contain the squash bugs or what kind of tomatoes make the best sauce. I am out in my garden most days in the summer, planting and weeding and pruning and harvesting. In the fall, with the help of the local yeasts and bacteria, I ferment the apples and cabbage into cider and sauerkraut.

I ask my patients who worry about yeast or parasites how much time they spend outside, whether or not they have pets, if they use antimicrobial soaps on their body or pesticides on their lawn. Some of them go along with me, but many more are impatient. They have been told so often that medicine has a pill for everything that they think I am just holding out on them. I wish I could prescribe instead just a few weeks of my grandmother's early twentieth-century lifestyle.

We've learned a lot about the microbiome in the past ten years, enough to turn the germ theory on its head, but there's still so much unknown. Although we have coined the term *dysbiosis* to describe a disordered microbiome, we still don't know how to recognize it in patients, what causes it, or how to fix it. How can we safely provide the challenges our immune system needs to develop while still protecting ourselves from serious illness and death? It will take a tremendous paradigm shift in how we think about our own body and how we conduct research to understand this complex system and to learn new ways of healing and nurturing our natural resilience, ways that might go against much that medicine has taught in the past 150 years. We will need evolutionary biologists, ecologists, healthcare providers, anthropologists, and clinical researchers working together, understanding that we are in a web with all other living things. Together, we must look critically at the forces pulling that web apart, as well as better understand the forces that hold it together.

Once we recognize our own bodies as ecosystems, we begin to see mesh-like networks of connection and communication everywhere we look, interlocking together with no boundaries. When we open our mind to the concept, it's easy to zoom out to look at the whole of Earth in an entirely new way, as an intricate, interconnected network of complex systems, or even as an organism, a holobiont itself, which makes humans and other living creatures part of Earth's microbiome.

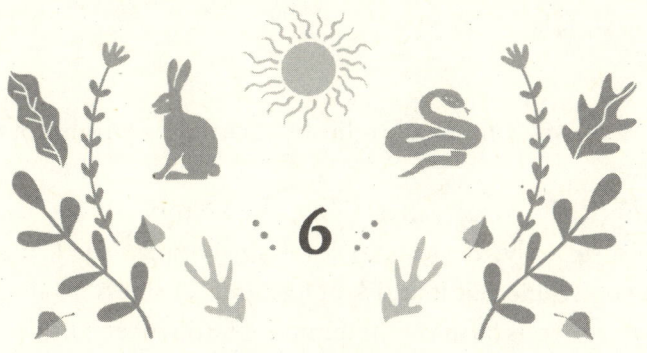

6

Gaia's Biome

We should be the heart and the mind of the earth, not its malady.

—JAMES LOVELOCK

My hometown of Toledo, Ohio, may not be the first place that springs to mind when one thinks of hotbeds of environmental radicalism, but in 2019 Toledo's citizens joined a revolutionary global movement. They passed a ballot initiative recognizing the legal personhood of a body of water—the "Lake Erie Bill of Rights." The amendment to the city's charter recognized "irrevocable rights for the Lake Erie Ecosystem to exist, flourish and naturally evolve, [and] a right to a healthy environment for the residents of Toledo [. . .], which elevates the rights of the community and its natural environment over powers claimed by certain corporations." Toledoans passed the measure in a creative attempt to address repeated threats to the environment and human health stemming from worsening contamination of the lake. Most dramatically, for three days in 2014, 400,000 people were unable to drink tap water due to the presence of toxins from a dangerous algae bloom. Activist Markie Miller of Toledoans for Safe Water told the press, "We've been using the same laws for decades to try and protect Lake Erie. They're clearly not working. Beginning today, with this historic vote, the people of Toledo and our allies are ushering in a new era of environmental rights by securing the rights of the Great Lake Erie."[1]

In politically conservative Ohio, the victory for the lake's rights was, unfortunately, fleeting. A local agribusiness sued, maintaining that the law would put it at risk of losing its business if someone were to file suit about its farm runoff dumping fertilizer and other chemicals into the lake. The court decided the law was too vague and that only the state had the power to pass regulations affecting the lake, and in doing so overruled the will of the citizens of Toledo.

Despite this setback, the movement to recognize the rights of nature is gaining ground across the globe. The contention that ecosystems have rights that extend beyond their possible uses by humans is a distinct shift away from the anthropocentrism that has dominated our relationship with nature, even within the environmental movement. As Gwendolyn Gordon explains in her 2017 article "Environmental Personhood," "Over time, the focus of legal and scholarly attention to the protection of nature has moved from being entirely focused on human interests in exploiting nature, to protecting nature for future human generations, to conceptions that allow for nature to be protected as intrinsically valuable."[2]

The idea that natural entities and ecosystems have intrinsic rights is resonant with common Indigenous worldviews that all living things have their own inherent value and are interrelated with humans as family, like the Andean concept of Pachamama, which literally translates as "Mother Earth" or "World Mother." She is seen as the originator and protector of all life and the mother of both the sun and moon gods. It is not surprising that the Andean nation of Ecuador, home to a large Indigenous population, became the first country to recognize the rights of nature in 2008, calling the constitutional provision the "Rights of Pachamama." The law gave standing to any citizen to "call upon public authorities to enforce the Rights of Nature" and recognized nature's right to "integral respect for its existence and for the maintenance and regeneration of its life cycles, structure, functions and evolutionary processes."[3]

Since that time, many other governments and courts have followed Ecuador's lead and enshrined the rights of nature. The Yurok Tribe of Northern California declared rights for the Klamath River in 2019 after years of low river flows had decimated salmon runs.[4] Now four dams have been removed, releasing the river from its human-made shackles and allowing it to run free—to the great benefit of the salmon, as well as surrounding ecosystems. The White Earth Nation in Minnesota adopted the Rights of Manoomin in 2018, recognizing the legal personhood of wild rice. It was the first known law encoded anywhere recognizing the rights of a plant.[5] In 2017 the New Zealand parliament protected the Whanganui River by granting it rights and also appointing two guardians to represent it, one from the government and one chosen by the Māori peoples. A 2016 court decision in Colombia acknowledged that the Rio Atrato, in the Pacific coast state of Choco, is its own entity with legal rights to protection, conservation, maintenance, and restoration. Like New Zealand, Colombia appointed guardians of the river to represent it, one from the government and one from local communities.

The idea that nature can be seen as a "person" may seem like a new age concept, but it has ancient roots. Many Indigenous cultures and religions viewed the earth itself as a conscious entity, the primal mother of all life. In addition being called Pachamama by the people of the Andes, she is known as Atabey by the Taino, the original people of the Caribbean islands; Akna by Mayans; It Bunoo by Indigenous people of northwest India, Bhutan, Nepal, and Tibet; Papatūānuku by Māori, and just Papa by original Hawaiians; Tatéi Yurianaka by the Huichol people who live still in Jalisco, Mexico; and Máttaráhkká by the Sámi of Scandinavia. Almost every Indigenous culture has some form of this concept. The view of the earth as a sentient being isn't just a religious or spiritual one, though; it's also supported by science.

The Gaia Hypothesis

In the 1960s, scientist James Lovelock was asked to collaborate with a team of NASA scientists to devise a way of determining whether a planet might foster life. Lovelock looked at the balance of gases in the atmospheres of Earth, Mars, and Venus, including the way their equilibrium changed over time. He quickly saw that high carbon dioxide levels on dead planets were static and unchanging. In contrast, Earth's balance of oxygen, carbon dioxide, and other compounds fluctuated in perfect rhythms to support existing life-forms. It looked more like a single organism's respiratory or circulatory system, with the gases dynamically flowing back and forth between states in ways that were unexplainable unless the interplay of all life on the planet was factored into the equation.

What Lovelock discovered in his work with NASA led him to posit that the Earth itself is one gigantic self-regulating ecosystem. His neighbor at the time, the novelist William Golding, suggested the poetic name the Gaia hypothesis, after the Greek Earth goddess and grandmother of Zeus. The theory proposed that living and nonliving parts of Earth form complex, interconnected systems that respond to changing conditions and evolve symbiotically over time, much as individual organisms do, and that these systems are predisposed to encourage and foster life. The emerging picture of Earth was one of a cohesive, integrated system, with many of the features of other life-forms. It was dynamic, interconnected, ever-changing, adaptable, and seemingly responding to some underlying operating system. In other words, Earth was alive and could even be considered sentient.

The idea was a revolutionary change from previous conceptions. As ecologist Stephan Harding describes it, prior to Lovelock's hypothesis "the Earth was thought of as a dead ball of rock with a thin smear of life on its surface, that didn't have any influence over what the composition of the surface looked like."[6] The living beings on Earth were considered passive passengers, and the tendencies of organisms and ecosystems were thought to resemble the mechanistic and predictable workings of a computer or a clock. Lovelock was suggesting that the whole earth itself was a living system, that it favored conditions that created life, and that it was ever evolving in response to the needs of that life force.

Although many of Lovelock's theories supporting the idea that Earth is a series of interdependent, evolving ecosystems have now been mainstreamed into the fields of biology, climatology, and ecology, they were extremely controversial at best, or considered anti-scientific anthropomorphism at worst, when first presented in the 1970s. The Gaia principle is the opposite of the religious view that nature was created to serve and be exploited by humans. It painted a picture of Earth as a living, breathing organism with its own priorities that have little to do with the parochial interests of *Homo sapiens*. Science is just now catching up with the ancient views many Indigenous cultures intuitively knew and have long held. Nature is a life force that connects every living being and even nonliving entities.

If Earth itself is best seen as a massively intricate organism, then it is not at all surprising that there are direct connections between clouds and algae, or between trees and microbes in the soil and rainfall. Nature is intelligent. The systems that regulate the earth and keep it inhabitable are not all known to us, like an invisible net that supports all living things. We can see some of the threads of the net, but many are not evident until they are out of balance or gone. Our net is fraying, and every strand we cut, every species extinguished, every rainforest burned, every river sucked dry, every additional ton of carbon dioxide pumped into the atmosphere threatens the integrity of the system and its ability to sustain life's diversity. How many cuts before the net is no longer reparable? How long before we overwhelm the inherent regulatory feedback mechanisms and cause the system to reset itself? We know from previous catastrophes—the resets can take millions of years.

In this view of the world, we are just one of many species interacting with others in an intricate, symbiotic, mesh-like web. On a universal scale, humans can be seen as a part of Gaia's biome, where we are one of many organisms interacting together. Much like the way our own microbiome functions, we can either contribute to Earth's overall well-being, or we can be the root cause of disease and dysfunction. Over the past few centuries, humankind has fallen mostly into the latter category. Our current predicament of human-made global warming, with its attendant hurricanes, wildfires, droughts, and floods, could be compared to a person with a fever, as if Gaia is already trying to eliminate an offending virus.

Our Role in Nature's Mesh of Life

It wasn't always this way. In the history of humanoids on Earth, going back hundreds of thousands of years, we have played many roles, sometimes destroyer, but often cultivator. With beavers, wolves and salmon, *Homo sapiens* is one of many keystone species in the arch of life, the species that many others depend on for their survival.

From early in our evolution, humans have had a profound impact on our surroundings. Even before the agricultural revolution, we were using fire to clear forests and create more favorable pasturelands to benefit the large grazers we depended on for food. In parts of the Rocky Mountains, humans may have herded plains buffalo into the mountains and "corralled" them in canyons, to be easily hunted when needed.[7] In the Amazon rainforest, humans used compost and charcoal to create thousands of acres of cultivatable land, called terra preta. The rich soil in these fertile "islands" is as deep as two meters and may cover 10 percent of the Amazon basin. People intentionally and methodically created conditions to encourage the spread of plants that were useful to them, thereby altering the entire ecosystem.[8]

Rediscovering the Lessons of Reciprocity

Lamentably, countless human cultures from which we might have learned important lessons of reciprocity between man and nature were wiped out by plague and destruction before they could be understood. Diseases carried across the globe by European colonists were a holocaust for Indigenous people, killing up to 90 percent of the population of the Americas. We now rely on storytellers and oral historians, along with archaeologists and anthropologists, to piece together lessons from fragments left behind. We can only wonder about the vast swaths of knowledge lost forever.

Despite humankind's wanton destruction, intentional and unintentional, against both nature and Indigenous peoples, some pockets of wisdom have been passed down from the ancestors—beacons that can point us to a different path, a way to live sustainably with nature. The collection of islands we know today as Hawai'i sits in an isolated patch of the Pacific, far from other landmasses, and subsequently was populated both by Polynesian settlers and European colonists much later than most of the world. Polynesians likely did not set up permanent villages until around 1000 CE. The nefarious Captain Cook was the first European to set foot on the islands in 1778. The first Hawai'ians organized themselves in a loose hierarchy, with watersheds forming the primary political divisions. Each chief oversaw a wedge-shaped area, called an ahupua'a, that stretched from mountaintops to the sea and included many ecosystems and a built-in water purification and irrigation system. Unlike in European feudal hierarchies, however, humans could not own the land; that was the provenance of the gods alone. Like the gods, the land was considered immortal and holy, and humans had the duty and privilege to care for it. There is even a Hawai'ian word for this kind of reciprocal relationship with the earth and other beings: kuleana. It describes a shared responsibility between two entities—people, other beings, or the earth itself—to care for and provide for each other.

In each ahupua'a, Hawai'ians practiced a complex form of conservation and land management that can still be seen today. The pristine highlands were traditionally off-limits to all but a few shamans, the bird hunters, charged with gathering brightly colored feathers for ceremonial robes. It was forbidden to cut down trees or disturb other fauna in these uplands, which were the origin of precious headwaters. The forested mountainsides retain and purify rainwater and prevent erosion, mitigating the effects of drought. Streams and rivers were revered and managed for crop irrigation, drinking water, and, nearer to the seashore, an intricate system of fishponds and aquaculture.

Everything was meticulously organized. Homes were built on rocky ground, preserving the best land for agriculture. Canals were created similar to the northern New Mexico acequia system. Land was terraced to retain water, with some crops reserved for irrigated land and some for wetter areas that needed only rainwater to sustain them. Even in the sea, fishing zones were assigned to specific communities, and at certain times of year fishing was prohibited for all. The Lima-huli Valley, one of the few intact ahupua'a remaining today, contains one of only two streams on Kauai where all five native species of fish can still be found; and the valley's higher mountaintops retain much more of their biodiversity than the areas that have been subdivided and developed without regard for the preserving the natural landscape.[9]

Forgetting Our Interdependence

Biologists characterize interspecies relationships into several categories: *mutual*, where both species benefit; *commensal*, where one benefits and the other is neither helped nor harmed; and *parasitic*, where one is helped at the expense of the other. While we cannot know for certain the magnitude of the influence that *Homo sapiens* had on the natural world prior to the modern era, the archaeological evidence seems to support that we acted more often in mutual or commensal ways. Our conversion from an often benign or beneficial to a mostly harmful relationship with Gaia has happened in just the past few hundred years, a nanosecond in geological time. In that short period, our technological ability to destroy outstripped our intellectual ability to understand the importance of what we are losing.

In the West, the loss of a reciprocity ethic with other beings—the philosophical shift to thinking humans are above nature—combined with the rise of capitalism to create a perfect formula for humankind's arrogant and extractive treatment of Earth. The Industrial Revolution gave us the tools and motivation to reap natural resources without regard—to clear forests, strip-mine mountaintops, and contaminate vast swaths of oceans, rivers, and land. Because most humans have become disconnected from our environment, we ignore the degradation until it's either literally killing us or we've lost something beautiful and irreplaceable. In recent years, we have been bombarded with dire reports documenting dramatic declines in the natural world and predicting more. A global study on insect populations cited habitat losses from agriculture along with the use of agrochemical pollutants and climate change as drivers for the decline in insect populations worldwide.[10] The researchers found that 40 percent of insect species are threatened with extinction. Another analysis released a few months later found that there are 3 billion fewer birds in North America compared to 1970, representing a 30 percent loss. The authors of the study called it "a staggering loss that suggests the very fabric of North America's ecosystem is unraveling."[11] Habitat encroachment by humans and pesticide use were cited as the culprits. Birds and insects are vital to the health of habitats; they serve as pollinators, fertilizers, and food for animals up and down the food chain. These two reports, among many others with similarly dire findings, signal the beginning of ecosystem collapse. One conservationist called it "the loss of nature."[12]

We are losing plants and animals at an astonishing rate. According to a 2019 United Nations report, the loss of over 1 million species is imminent, due to direct human encroachment on habitat and indirect human influence through climate change. The chair of the group that conducted the assessment, Sir Robert Watson, said, "We are eroding the very foundations of economies, livelihoods, food security, health and quality of life worldwide."[13] Many of the species at risk will have come and gone from the earth unknown to us. Of the estimated 8 million to 9 million species on earth, we have "discovered" only 1.3 million, or 14 percent.[14] Creatures are being extinguished faster than we can name them. Sixty percent of the world's wildlife has been wiped out since 1970. It's hard to stop the dominoes from falling once the chain reaction starts, and in this case many of the dominoes are invisible to us until they've already toppled. We are not sure what will happen, for example, if the coral reefs collapse en masse, or insects disappear. Which domino, if it falls, will cause the whole system to come tumbling down? Where is the tipping point?

In anticipation of the coming catastrophe, some of the uber-wealthy seem to have already given up on planet Earth in favor of finding somewhere else we could start anew. Billionaires try to one-up each other building the fastest, most powerful rocket as if they're playing some children's game. One of these, Elon Musk, believes that "for us to have a future that's exciting and inspiring, it has to be one where we're a space-bearing civilization." Musk seems ready to give up on this planet and its life-support system that has evolved perfectly to support humans and other beings over the course of millions of years. He thinks he can do better in just a few decades. He's dedicating his prodigious fortune to the goal of creating a self-sustaining city on Mars before 2050. He plans to "bring the animals and creatures of Earth there, sort of like a futuristic Noah's ark. We'll bring more than two, though—it's a little weird if there's only two."[15] Musk and his fellow disconnected billionaires don't understand that replicating the whole intricate symphony that connects and supports all life isn't so simple. Like rich, bored children, they can't see the wonder right in front of them. Imagine if they would invest their fortunes instead in saving *our* planet, with all its beauty and mystery and complex life-giving systems that have evolved over eons.

Will humankind take the steps necessary to rediscover our interdependence with the natural world? Or will we march forward on our current path until the earth becomes uninhabitable for *Homo sapiens* and thousands of other species? As part of Earth's microbiome, humankind has become a dangerous infection threatening Gaia's well-being. Some damage is most certainly irrevocable. Although we cannot bring back extinct species (probably) or melted glaciers, there still may be time to chart a new path. It will require a stark societal shift and acting from a place of consciousness of our embeddedness in and dependence on the natural world. Instead of using technology to exploit and destroy Earth, or to leave it entirely, can we find our way back to a way of life that benefits our home biosphere and the other living beings we share it with? Whatever course we choose, most people believe Gaia will regenerate, as she has done at least five times before. The questions are: Will it take a few centuries, or a few millennia? And will it be with us or without us? The answers will largely depend on the choices we make in the next few decades, and whether we can see ourselves as an integrated part of Gaia's biome, rather than separate from and above "nature."

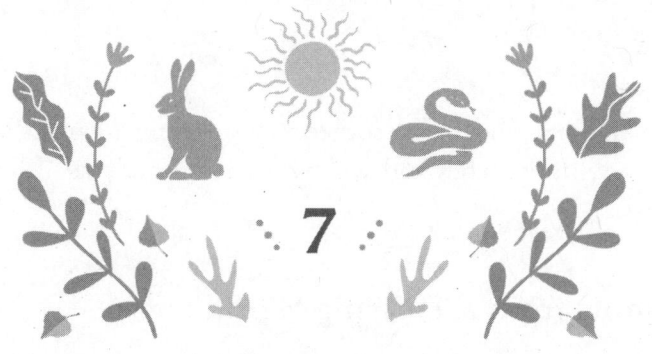

We Are Nature

An awareness of nature is not . . . a sentimental or spiritual
practice, but a profoundly realistic one—a way of binding
ourselves to the simple truth that human beings depend
on ecological systems for our survival.

—J. B. MACKINNON, *THE ONCE AND FUTURE WORLD*

Some of my strongest childhood memories are snapshots of the natural
world.

A constellation of lightning bugs rises from the forest floor in the
dusk, glowing and flashing their secret code to each other on a humid
Midwestern summer full-moon night. My brother and I scamper
through the brush, trying to catch a few in mason jars for makeshift
wild lanterns.

A few weeks after the last frost in spring, the ditch in front of our
house is suddenly teeming with tadpoles. I scoop out a few and put
them in a green plastic tub in the front yard so I can watch their meta-
morphosis over the coming days, mystified when they vanish from
one day to the next.

With only my black lab, Pepper, for company, I set out to explore
neighborhood creek beds and rivers, keeping an eye out for deer,

raccoon, rabbits, and birds, sometimes stopping to make a lean-to hideaway with branches and yellow leaves recently shed by almost-bare trees.

Snapshots from a Thriving World

I grew up along the shores of Lake Erie, near the rust-belt cities of Buffalo, Cleveland, and Toledo. Despite money being tight and a lot of moving around to chase jobs, my parents always made sure we landed in a neighborhood with good schools and plenty of places to play and explore. Every summer, our low-budget vacation was a long camping trip. The Smoky Mountains, the Adirondacks, and Luding-ton Park in the sand dunes of western Michigan were among my favorite destinations.

During one trip to the Finger Lakes in upstate New York when I was about nine, I was very excited by the prospect that we might see a bear. I remember being awakened by my father in the middle of the night. "Wendy, do you want to see that bear?" Groggily, I propped myself up and looked out the screen window of our musty canvas tent to see a very contented bear tearing open our cooler, smashing eggs into his mouth, and washing them down with a gallon of milk. I watched with fascination and fear.

In a time beyond the reach of my memory, when I was two, we went to Algonquin Park in Canada during the season of unrelenting black flies. Mom tells me that they seemed particularly attracted to my young flesh and I spent much of the vacation with blood dripping down my face and arms like a scene from some horror movie, but I didn't seem to mind much.

The natural world nourished me, and I guess I nourished it a bit too. I found solace in the wild spaces around me, like a trusted friend I could always count on. When I was feeling lonely or sad, which was fairly often as we moved so frequently, the woods and the creeks and the creatures that inhabited them were my companions and my touchstone. It's no surprise that my childhood connection to nature developed into an adult love and appreciation of all the living things we share the planet with. In my post-childhood life, I've deepened that connection with more exploration, learning, and pursuits like birding, gardening, hiking, wildcrafting, and foraging, following in the footsteps of my ancestors.

An Essential Vitamin: Nature's Wild Places

Although I was unaware of it at the time, my early connection to nature likely contributed to the good health I've enjoyed as an adult. Children with more exposure to green spaces have a lower incidence of mental health problems, are more physically active, and less likely to be overweight. They are also less likely to have chronic immune problems like asthma and eczema. Kids and adults with regular exposure to nature learn better, are less stressed, and are more focused. Time in the natural world can be especially healing for people with histories of trauma or attention deficit disorder. And the more biodiverse our natural spaces are, the more all these effects are enhanced. It turns out that nature, in all its complexity, may be essential for optimal mental and physical health.

A study by the London School of Economics designed to determine the conditions that create a sense of happiness and contentment in humans across the globe used an app called Mappiness that randomly pings participants who have voluntarily downloaded it. Individuals are asked to record their feelings in the moment and describe their surroundings and situation. Early findings from the research showed that participants were significantly happier in outdoor environments, even controlling for bad weather and if they were with companions or alone.[1]

Although we may be happiest outdoors in nature, the EPA estimates that average American spends about 90 percent of their life indoors.[2] Despite what we may desire, our lifestyles and culture aren't conducive to being in nature much. Still, most of us crave it, consciously or unconsciously. Research shows that time outside alleviates stress and contributes to an overall sense of well-being. One study even quantified the optimum dose of nature at about 200–300 minutes per week, with no harms found from overdosing.[3] Time in green places doesn't just subjectively make us feel better, but it also has measurable physiologic effects like lowering blood pressure, improving sleep and cognitive function, and even reducing risk of cardiovascular disease, depression, and anxiety.[4] Even people who cannot physically go outside, like inpatients in hospitals, benefit from exposure to the natural world. Patients whose window looked out on green space rather than a brick wall were shown to recover faster from surgery and need less pain medication.[5]

Wild places enhance our individual well-being, but they are also critical for our continued collective existence as a species. Well-functioning ecosystems, be they in forests or deserts or oceans, serve to regenerate soils and make agriculture possible, filter and store water, clean the air, and store carbon to mitigate global warming. Even in cities and urban areas, the presence and integration of nature is increasingly critical to stave off the devastating effects of climate change. Neighborhoods with more trees can be as much as 10–20 degrees Fahrenheit cooler than those with no tree cover. That differential literally means the difference between life and death during the increasingly intense summertime heat waves now commonplace in most North American and European cities.[6]

Dangerously, some people try to boil down nature simply to the quantifiable benefits it can offer humans, putting an economic value, a price tag, on "ecosystem services"—those very tangible things that the natural world provides us. The thinking goes that if environmentalists have been only marginally successful at arguing for the preservation of nature merely for nature's sake, they would do better by putting their arguments into the cold economic terms that businesspeople and politicians seem to understand better. But the very concept that nature is exclusively there to serve us is part of the problem—it leads us to value only those things that can be bought and sold. It reduces nature to less than a sum of its parts, then sells those parts off as commodities in the same capitalist marketplace tearing nature apart. It's akin to a machine view of the natural world. When we sell the idea of nature as a commodity, those parts that cannot be commodified become worthless to the machine, and interest in learning about the natural world for its own sake fades.

Lost Words, Lost Places, Lost Memories

A hundred-plus years ago, most people knew the names of the prevalent plants and trees that grew in their neighborhoods, on their farms, and in their local parks. Over the past couple of centuries, the ability to name even common species of trees, plants, birds, and fish has eroded so much that the few people who are still able to do so are seen as oddities. "Plant blindness" has become a problem even in academia, where university curricula have shifted from unpopular courses of study like plant ecology to more lucrative fields like molecular biology. Students are following the money and eschewing majors that won't lead to sustainable careers once they graduate. The Next Generation Science Standards, part of the Common Core effort to standardize K–12 science curricula, are notable for their lack of emphasis on the study of nature. The shift to case study–style integrated classes might facilitate teaching about climate change and evolution, but some important things will be lost. I trace the roots of my interest in medicine back to Mr. Kocher's tenth-grade biology class, where we dissected earthworms and starfish and drew the outsides and insides of plants and animals to better understand their classifications into kingdoms, phyla, orders, and families. Today's business- and career-focused schools and universities have little time to delve into arcane pursuits like these.

The loss of words is reflected in our classrooms, our literature, and our dictionaries. A study by cognitive psychologists Douglas Medin and Phillip Wolff looked at the frequency of use of three categories of tree names in the English language: first the generic *tree*, then the slightly more specific *oak* or *spruce*, and finally the most precise *gambel oak* or *blue spruce*. They found that from the 1500s to the 1800s, tree terms proliferated and became increasingly more specific, but then noted a marked decline after the Industrial Revolution in the nineteenth and twentieth centuries.[7] In 2007, the *Oxford Junior Dictionary* eliminated many words naming things in the natural world, like *wren*, *moss*, and *bluebell*, in favor of words more useful in our human and technology-centered world, like *celebrity*, *voicemail*, and *broadband*.

We create names and vocabulary for what holds our attention, and we forget the words for things that no longer interest us. Language follows our senses. When we replace the specific name *white ash* or *American chestnut* or *piñon pine* with the generic *tree* or even *pine tree*, all trees become an undistinguishable mass, and the decline or loss of a certain species passes unnoticed. When we don't care enough about something to even name it, we are unlikely to feel relationship with it, or acknowledge that it may have any effect on our life. Who will miss the silvery minnow or the spotted owl or even the red panda, if one fish or bird or furry animal is interchangeable with another? The loss of words mirrors not only our disconnection from nature but also the loss of the actual biodiversity. Far fewer children born today will have the experiences of capturing lightning bugs, gathering tadpoles, or seeing bears in the wild. They will experience what they will call nature, but it will be much different from the nature I knew right outside my front door on the outskirts of Toledo.

As we lose biodiversity and even the words for describing it, we also lose the memory itself of how rich and full the world was just a few decades ago. Each generation sees its environment as the baseline. It's hard to convey to people born twenty years ago what fifty years ago was like. Even older people forget how abundant nature was in our own childhood. The phenomenon is known to naturalists and ecologists as the "shifting baseline." Canadian naturalist J. B. MacKinnon writes, "Our own ancestors handed down a degraded globe, and we accepted that inheritance as the normal state of things. As our parents and grandparents did before us, we go about our lives in the midst of an ecological catastrophe that is well underway."[8] If I go back to those suburbs where I grew up, there are no more forests brimming with lightning bugs, no more tadpole-filled ditches. They exist only in my memory. When I am gone, those memories will perish with me. The few scientists who study natural history know we now live in a "10 percent world," surrounded by just a fraction of the wildness that once existed. The rest of us walk in a fog of amnesia.

Refuge vs. Rewild

One response to this massive global tragedy unfolding before our eyes has been to try to fence off some "pristine" areas while the rest is fair game for pillaging. Wilderness is relegated to a patchwork of national parks, monuments, and places that are, for the most part, inhospitable to human settlement. Most of these are places assumed to be devoid of extractive resources—until some valuable commodity is found within their boundaries. Almost 30 percent of the United States is federal public land, much managed primarily to bene-fit humans for grazing, logging, mining, hunting, and recreation. Under 5 percent of the total US landmass is preserved as wildlife refuges, the highest level of protection. More than 80 percent of those wilds are in Alaska, with 19 million acres in Arctic National Wildlife Refuge, currently the subject of much dispute as we seek ever more sources of fossil fuels to feed our dependence. The rest of these pieces of land are scattered, small, and isolated from each other. Like broken shards of pottery spread across the landscape, each one might be beautiful, but they make so much more sense and are more functional when they are joined together.

Attempts to preserve disparate wild areas have made it clear that ecosystems don't flourish in isolation. In the late 1960s, while studying the nature of biodiversity on actual islands, biologists E. O. Wilson and Robert MacArthur established the theory of island biogeography. They determined that the size of an island is directly related to the number of life-forms it can maintain. The larger an island, the more diverse it can be. Later, the theory was found to hold true for other types of human-made islands, like national parks and wildlife refuges hemmed in by human habitation. When we create artificial islands of wilderness and cut them off from the natural historic ranges of the animals who inhabit them, the number of species begins to dwindle.

The disappearance of wolves from Yellowstone Park by the 1940s is a famous case in point. When the park was established in 1872, gray wolves were already in decline, suffering from the encroachment of agricultural land. As more humans moved west, the wolf was seen as a greater menace. Deprived of their natural prey, the wolves turned to settlers' livestock. Between 1914 and 1926, 136 wolves were killed inside the park, and many more outside the park, by settlers and by the stewards of the park themselves. The wolves were not the only species targeted. Populations of all large predators were decimated, including those of cougars, bears, and coyotes, but the wolves were eliminated completely. The park managers wanted not only to protect the cows and sheep grazing near the park but also to favor more "desirable" wild animals like elk and deer.

In the decades that followed the eradication of the wolves, elk and deer populations exploded. Forested areas declined as all the new saplings were devoured by the ungulates, and no young trees could survive long enough to replace the older ones. Beavers couldn't find enough nourishment so their populations dropped. That set off a cascade of other losses—of fishes, amphibians, and the animals that preyed on them—as the aquatic environments they needed to survive diminished. Finally, in 1995, wolves were reintroduced, but not without great and sustained controversy from area ranchers. In the decades since, beavers and forests and wetlands have started to return, along with many other species that depended on them. The effect of this kind of "rewilding" is called a trophic cascade, when the reintroduction of one keystone species transforms the entire ecosystem, making it much more diverse, healthy, and resilient.

Following the experience in Yellowstone, rewilding projects have caught on in regions across the globe. Mexican wolves, which became extinct in the wild by the 1980s, were brought back to New Mexico and Arizona in 1998. Plans are underway to reintroduce large grazing herbivores and predators like European lynx to several remote areas in Europe. Conservation planning now routinely includes the creation of corridors so that wildlife can safely migrate and travel in search of food and homes, or escape to safer ground in case of natural disasters like droughts or floods or wildfires. These pathways allow populations to grow, and in the age of accelerating climate change, linkages between wild areas are more critical than ever.

All these projects have their detractors, and many, like the Yellowstone wolf project, continue to be mired in conflict and controversy. Opponents of rewilding cite dangers to livestock and to humans. On the other hand, proponents argue that the alternative to rewilding is to continue to let our ecosystems degrade, to let our 10 percent world turn into a 5 percent world and finally a 1 percent world. The ranchers and farmers are concerned about the risks of nature to their livelihoods, but what of the risks of the lack of nature? We may continue to adapt to the losses, but what is the price?

Ultimately, rewilding efforts will fall short if we can't rewild our own relationship with nature. Conservation efforts that pretend humans don't exist, or exclude sustainable relationships between humans and the land, are doomed to fail. Conversely, if humans persist in demanding that all risk be removed from the natural world, or that our role as nature's overlords means we have the right to take and kill anything at any time, we will destroy what makes wilderness wild. As human population continues to grow and spread, the lands where wildlife and people both claim homes and habitat also increases. A recent study predicted that the areas of human–wildlife overlap will increase over about 57 percent of Earth's land.[9] Finding new ways to coexist peacefully is critical for the survival of all beings.

Indigenous people all over the earth have negotiated relationships with wilderness and come up with numerous different answers to problems of conservation and rewilding. These solutions usually include space for healthy human interdependence with the natural world. Currently, the Pyramid Lake Paiute Tribe is reintroducing bighorn sheep on their lands in California. The species plays an important role in their culture for food, pelts, and ceremonial uses but hasn't been available to them for over a hundred years. The large grazers will help revitalize the land by nourishing soils, distributing seeds, and controlling underbrush. The Paiute plan to rewild the land also will revitalize their own cultural practices, so the two species can return to their symbiotic relationship of ancient times.

The Maasai of eastern Africa who make their livelihood as cattle herders have had a mutually respectful relationship with lions for hundreds of years. The lions sometimes take livestock and the Maasai hunt lions, mostly ceremonially. Historically, killing a lion on a hunt was and important rite of passage for young Maasai men. Their relationship is one of respect and understanding. The hunting process was highly ritualized and has many rules, for example that female lions should not be killed, or that no lions should be killed in times of drought, or by snares or traps. The Maasai recognized the lion's role in the ecosystem, keeping other predators in check, while they also took steps to reduce the inherent risk in coexisting with a predator. The fact that the 20 percent of the Earth's surface still under Indigenous stewardship contains the most biodiverse areas where humans and wildlife can coexist is not a coincidence.[10]

Most of us have unrealistic expectations of risk in nature. We want to be able to dip our toes in its pleasure while being shielded from all harm. Of course, our human-made world has risks too, but mostly we tolerate them because of the benefits modern conveniences bring. To the extent possible, we protect ourselves by wearing seatbelts in cars or deploying air traffic control systems to prevent plane crashes. We practice what is called harm reduction in public health. We know drinking alcohol can be risky, so we designate a driver and limit our consumption. When we decide that something is necessary to our quality of life, even if it is sometimes dangerous, we find ways to minimize harm. If we want to reap the benefits that revitalizing our ecosystems can bring, we must think of ways to practice harm reduction for both humans and other beings in wild places. These methods aren't hard to employ; we have ways to protect livestock without killing wolves, for example, but they might require shifting grazing practices or more investment for costlier non-wolf-lethal solutions.

Reintegrating on a Smaller Scale

Rewilding projects don't need to be as grandiose as bringing wolves back to Yellowstone, lynx back to Scotland, or bighorn sheep to Pyramid Lake. In 2016 a retired teacher scuba diving off the coast of Southern California discovered a small colony of seahorses and has been visiting and protecting them ever since. A couple in England bought twenty acres of over-farmed land, then restored its marshes and wetlands, and watched as the birds, animals, and plant life quickly returned. Famed Brazilian photographer Sebastião Salgado moved back to his family's deforested farm and found less than 0.5 percent of the land was still tree-covered. He and his wife decided to reforest the homestead, planting two million trees. Twenty years later the saplings have grown into a forest, nurturing a diverse ecosystem where before was barren, degraded farmland. Many people have recently redis-covered regenerative agricultural practices employed by Indigenous people for eons and are creating farms that are useful to both humans and our wild kin.

Closer to Home

On my couple of acres, I've identified nearly 100 bird species, from turkey vultures and great horned owls to bushtits and ruby-crowned kinglets, including the blue heron and the mallard who fleetingly decided to explore my micro-pond. I often record the choruses of competing bird songs, wanting to remember the intricate overlap-ping melodies in years to come, never knowing if this might be the peak songbird year of my lifetime. In winter, the juncos and pine siskins flock to the feeders. Would I notice if their numbers were cut in half? In late summer, if I sit calmly by the pond for a long stretch, my patience will be rewarded by a glimpse of the shy green towhee taking a furtive sip of water, or a hermit thrush bathing, or a garter snake stalking its prey. I often carefully walk the whole yard, paying attention to new wildflowers and plants that have spontaneously appeared. On a recent foray I noted native desert four o'clocks, silver nightshade, and wild rye. Would it matter terribly if one these species was erased?

Living Together

Neither large-scale rewilding nor personal efforts to replace lawns with meadows will reverse our trajectory by themselves. For that, we will need to reimagine our relationship with Gaia and our place in the world of living things. We will have to relearn from the world's threatened Indigenous cultures how to live embedded in natural eco-systems, and we will have to adapt our lifestyles, our cities, and our homes in ways that invite nature to enter, and accept that although it's sometimes messy and chaotic, the benefits far outweigh the costs.

Trying to live symbiotically with wildlife isn't always easy. As I write this, I can hear the scratching overhead from a couple of fat rac-coons in the eaves of my roof, just waking up for their nocturnal prowl. They have so far evaded all attempts to lure them into the live trap or dissuade them from their choice of homestead. In spring, I will have to be vigilant to prevent the flickers from carving out my stucco walls for their nests. But there is also beauty and wonder. As I put the bird feed-ers out, before I can walk away, a flock of twenty bushtits descend like a mass of feathered pom-poms. They are unbothered as I watch them from less than an arm's length away. Just a few minutes ago I heard the coyotes howling and went outside for a better listen. I was rewarded to see a frisky pair frolicking in the snow a few feet beyond the porch. For all the messiness and inconvenience that comes from living enmeshed in nature, there are tenfold benefits to my well-being, my stress level, and even my microbiome and physical health.

Maybe if we could see these other creatures as beings much closer to us and lose our human superiority, it would be harder to think about destroying them. If we could see our wild brethren as kin, the sharp dividing line between the natural and the human worlds would start to blur. When we think of our whole ecosystem and all the important connections encompassed within, our ties to the natural world aren't the only consideration, however. Healthy relationships with other humans are just as important.

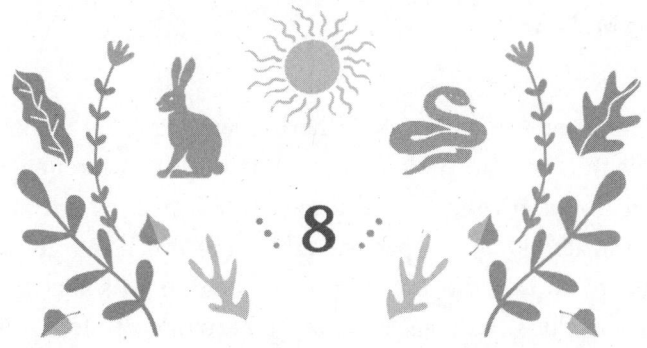

8

Humans Are Social Animals

Rarely, if ever, are any of us healed in isolation.
Healing is an act of communion.

—bell hooks

My dog Luca needs his people. Sometimes when guests are visiting, they'll take Luca for a walk to the arroyo near my house without me. Although he starts out excited to explore with new friends, invariably he shows up back at the house several minutes before the rest of the crew, running ahead as soon as he sees the trail that leads back over the hill between the arroyo and the dirt road, racing down the gravel driveway, then prancing back and forth excitedly in front of the windows as if to say, "I'm back, did you miss me? I missed you *a lot.*" By contrast, when he's out with me and his other pack-mate, Stella, he's content to hang with his family for as long as we amble along together. Like the wolves he descended from, and like so many other animals—birds and deer and javelinas and bees—Luca instinctively knows he needs his people to be healthy and survive.

We need our people too. Whether we realize it or not, we all have a lot in common with Luca. Public health researchers use scales of "social isolation" and "social integration" to study the ways community and family ties impact health. High social integration scores are given to those who are partnered, belong to social groups like churches or clubs, and have a strong network of close friends and family they can depend on. The research is clear—loneliness and disconnection are linked to significant mental and physical health problems including anxiety, depression, insomnia, dementia, heart disease and stroke, decreased immune function, suicide, and excessive drug and alcohol use.[1] As society becomes more socially disconnected, rates of these correlated maladies are on the rise.

Isolation and loneliness can be deadly—worse even than obesity, a sedentary lifestyle, or excessive drinking, the health issues we're warned about every day. Taken together, the research shows that living without close human connections increases mortality by up to 50 percent. Those with high degrees of social isolation can expect their lifespan to be shortened as much as if they smoked almost a pack of cigarettes a day.[2]

Given the dangers of aloneness and the benefits of trusted relationships, one would assume that the public health system would focus heavily on mitigating these risks, much as it does for similarly harmful factors like smoking or drinking or obesity. In reality, it's hard to find attention focused on community connections. In the United States, there are almost no campaigns to educate folks about the dangers of being alone and few public programs to help people suffering from loneliness connect with others. Quite the contrary, our culture extols the values of rugged individualism and "going it alone." When we see a colleague or a friend experience either success or failure, we credit (or blame) the individual, when there is always a backstory with a larger cast of characters.

Americans especially imagine themselves to be a nation of individual players, living and dying solely due to their own personal choices. As sociologist Robin M. Williams describes it, in the United

States "the ultimate source of action, meaning, and responsibility is the individual rather than the group."[3] Like our public health institutions, our healthcare system gives little consideration to the effects of communities and relationships on our health. To the contrary, a tacit assumption baked into the practice of Western medicine is that our patients' well-being is almost exclusively determined by their own specific beliefs and behaviors. Even the few classes in medical school about social determinants of health often seem to implicate individual behaviors as much as societal factors. The bulk of medical science, practice, and education reflects the erroneous conviction that the individual is the nidus of all responsibility. The belief affects everything, from the way we interview patients, to the way we construct our hospitals, to the remedies we prescribe.

Instead of seeing patients as they truly are, embedded in a web of relationships, most healthcare providers act as if patients exist in separate bubbles and focus almost exclusively on individual lifestyles and behaviors. Evidence paints a different picture; it shows that even those "behaviors" many doctors ascribe to patients' bad choices are largely determined by the social environment. Those with high social isolation scores are much more likely to have poor diets, drink too much, and smoke. Even though these activities may appear to be driven by personal choices, oftentimes they act more like contagions. Researchers found that when one individual in a family gained weight, others were more likely to follow suit. Patients who are surrounded by friends who are overweight are more likely to become overweight themselves. The closer the connection, the more likely that one person will "pass" obesity on to another.[4]

Like the underground fungal webs that serve as a network of communication between trees in a forest, the threads that bind us together and keep us healthy might not be so evident even to ourselves. They are hard to see when so much in our society supports the myth that each person is the sole architect of their own fate, and when billions of dollars are spent each year reinforcing this lie. In recent years the global "wellness industry" has grown twice as fast as the global economy, valued at over $5 trillion in 2022 and expected to grow to over $8 trillion by 2027.[5] Their many gurus promise if we just eat the right diet, do the right exercises, or take the right supplements, we can be slim and beautiful, banish our aches and pains, and cure our chronic illnesses. They promise fast and dramatic results via secret solutions or "one weird trick" easily obtained for a modest monthly subscription fee.

The delusion that we are just one diet or exercise program away from living our best life creates more misery than salvation. Every dollar spent on the newest fad propagates an illusion that our individual agency can be separated from our social milieu and commodifies our desires for connection and happiness. As a species, or as separate organisms, our well-being is inextricably bound up with our family and friends, our workplace, our community, our environment, and even the neighborhood where we reside. No one can change their lifestyle entirely on their own—we all require a network of support and connection. Escaping patterns that are engrained in and encouraged by our culture or society can be all but impossible unless the culture or society also changes. Whether we like it or not, we're all in this together. We may not all be in the same boat, but we are certainly all in the same ocean.

As individuals, we might find the challenge to change our culture or community even more daunting than changing our personal behavior. Policymakers and public health professionals are beginning to see the power of social connection and are grappling with how to create programs that address and overcome individual isolation on a population level. In 2018 Britain launched a major initiative to combat loneliness including a comprehensive public health strategy, public awareness campaigns, the development of national surveys and measures to track feelings of disconnection, and even the appointment of a "minister for loneliness." More than five years later, it's hard to see many concrete effects of these social interventions.[6] More people than ever are living alone, the COVID pandemic canceled most gatherings for several years, social media often replaces in-person interactions, and a worsening economic situation means there's less cash to spend on going out. The challenges to reigniting interdependence have been daunting. Before we give up hope, it may be helpful to look at other times and other cultures to better understand the building blocks of social connection.

The Roseto Effect

The story of Roseto, Pennsylvania, beautifully illustrates the overwhelming influence of culture and connection on human health. A physician working in Roseto in the 1960s noted to a colleague at a medical conference that despite high rates of smoking, drinking, and high-fat diets among his patients, he had diagnosed almost no heart disease for several years. In fact, he could not remember the last time one of his patients died from a heart attack. The town was settled by immigrants from Roseto, Italy, starting in the 1880s. From the early 1900s until the late 1970s, almost all the 1,600 inhabitants were descended from immigrants from this one small Italian mountain town. Their families had ties to each other going back centuries.

The two doctors decided to formally study the population and found that from 1954 to 1961, there were in fact no deaths from heart disease. The mortality rates for Roseto men over sixty-five were half that of the general US population. The subsequently dubbed "Roseto effect" was credited to the low stress engendered by a tight-knit community where everyone knew each other and helped each other, along with low rates of economic inequality. Those "individual" wellness factors like diet, smoking, and exercise didn't seem to matter so much in Roseto—community cohesiveness washed out their most detrimental effects.

A review of the Roseto data in 1992 looked at death certificates and other population-level data for the town and compared it to a neighboring town, Bangor, during the same period. The study confirmed a strikingly low mortality rate in Roseto that lasted almost 100 years after the first Italian immigrants settled there. During the years of lower mortality rates, roughly until 1965, the diet, smoking rates, and occupations were similar to those in Bangor. Roseto only lost its special advantage in the 1960s and 1970s. Researchers concluded that the major change in Roseto after 1960 was a loss of social cohesion.[7]

The "Americanization" of the population with all its attendant stressors, isolation, and inequalities began to encroach on the town in the turbulent 1960s and 1970s. By the 1990s, the rates of heart disease and mortality in Roseto had caught up with neighboring towns. A similar effect can be seen among recent immigrants in a phenomenon that has been dubbed the "Latino paradox." Despite being more socio-economically disadvantaged, recent immigrants from Latin America have health indicators, especially birth outcomes, on par with those of wealthy white Americans. The effect diminishes after a generation or two, as immigrants become more assimilated and also suffer the effects of living in a less healthy and more inequitable society.

Mistrustful and Stressed Out

The experience of Roseto's population isn't unique. Everywhere in the world, when social divisions and isolation deepen, levels of stress and anxiety increase, giving rise to higher rates of mental illness, suicides, and deaths related to alcohol, drugs, and tobacco, popularly called "deaths of despair." Although that term has been applied primarily to middle-aged, poor, non–Hispanic whites, mortality rates from these causes have been increasing in nearly all racial and ethnic groups, shortening life spans across the board.

For most of the past 100 years, life expectancies in the United States grew steadily. The gains began to flatten out in the early 2000s and then started to decline in 2015. In 2020, we experienced the steepest drop since World War II. Much of the 1.8 years lost in average life spans that year was due the COVID-19 pandemic, but deaths from heart disease, stroke and Alzheimer's disease also rose. Increases in rates of homicides, suicides, and drug overdoses have hit young people especially hard. The coronavirus epidemic disproportionately affected people of color, with Hispanics losing 3 years of life expectancy and Blacks 2.9 years, compared to a 1.2-year drop for non–Hispanic whites.[8]

Although the pandemic might be blamed for much of the decline through 2022, that doesn't account for the shortening of average lifespans in the prior years, or why they have flattened out across the globe, especially for disadvantaged populations. What is changing about our society that leads to so many early deaths? According to former US Surgeon General Vivek Murthy, there is a growing and largely unchecked epidemic of social disconnection in the United States—rates have doubled since the 1980s, and fewer people than ever report having a trusted close friend in their life.[9] The social isolation and physical distancing imposed by the COVID pandemic only exacerbated the problem.

In a vicious cycle, social isolation and loneliness beget more distrust and deeper withdrawal from society. Drs. John and Stephanie Cacioppo studied the neurological and cognitive effects of social disconnection for years. They found that people who describe themselves as lonely are more distrustful and twice as likely to imagine social threats around them, even keeping more physical space between themselves and loved ones at family gatherings. The lonely brain becomes increasingly hypervigilant and more likely to perceive rejection or interpersonal hostility in social interactions.[10] More and more disconnection creates a self-perpetuating cycle of societal divisions.

Although many countries have experienced a slowdown in lengthening life expectancies over the past few years, few have seen the steep declines of the United States. In 2020 only Russia had a larger drop. What is it about a country or a community that confers resiliency, or conversely, greater vulnerability when inevitable threats to health and longevity, like a global pandemic, come along?

Inequality Kills

Your zip code determines more about the length of your life than your genetic code. Maps of places with high rates of smoking, drinking, drug use, obesity, and social isolation overlap with areas of poverty and inequities. Stress caused by inequality, racism, and violence can blanket whole communities and give rise to both greater social disintegration and higher levels of many ills that impact the well-being of everyone living in the neighborhood. Oppression and marginalization perpetuate poor health, which in turn creates more trauma and stress, more illness and malaise, and the cycle continues. All the while, our healthcare system ignores these community attributes and puts the onus on individuals to "fix" problems that are actually systemic in nature. To obese patients we say, "Eat a healthier diet" or "Exercise more," ignoring the mountain of evidence that shows the stress of living in an unhealthy environment mostly overwhelms individual efforts to change behaviors.

The idea that poverty is unhealthy isn't new. For centuries now public health professionals have recognized the "diseases of the poor" and observed that those living at the bottom of the socioeconomic ladder suffer more illness and live shorter lives than those at the top. Interestingly, in the past fifty years, researchers began to notice there are exceptions to this rule. When studying the health effects of poverty, they saw unexpected patterns. In some places of relative poverty, populations were much healthier and had longer life expectancies than in wealthier areas.

In his 1999 book *Development as Freedom*, Nobel Prize–winning economist Amartya Sen pointed out places like Kerala state in India, Sri Lanka, and Costa Rica where inhabitants were healthier, longer-lived, and happier than in much wealthier countries. Sen and other researchers identified protective factors in these overall poorer-but-healthier regions related to greater social supports and equity. Places with smaller differences between rich and poor were more socially cohesive and had economic development policies that raised all boats equally rather than creating deeper divides. Social programs made sure everyone had access to essential resources like healthcare, housing, and education.[11]

In the United States, one of the first studies to consider social networks and their long-term effects on health and mortality started in 1964 in Alameda County, California, and continued for over thirty years. Researchers created a neighborhood social environment scale based on the level of commercial activity, overall socioeconomic status, the quality of housing, and other environmental factors. As expected, mortality rates were higher for those living in neighborhoods with lower social environment scores. The key finding, just like in Roseto, was behaviors didn't matter as much as addresses. The study controlled for independent risk factors like individual income level, education, race/ethnicity, smoking status, body mass index, and alcohol consumption, but still found significantly higher mortality risks among residents in low-score neighborhoods. Put another way: even fit, rich, highly educated, nonsmokers and nondrinkers living in neighborhoods with poor social environments are more likely to die younger than their counterparts in more well-off neighborhoods.[12]

The lesson may appear to be that it's preferable to be the poorest person in a rich neighborhood than the richest person in a poor neighborhood, but social cohesion doesn't necessarily get better as you go up the economic ladder, as anyone who has lived in a gated community with a homeowners' association can likely attest. A more important factor than overall socioeconomic status of a population seems to be the degree of inequality. In our capitalistic world, the gradients between rich and poor have grown starker almost everywhere in recent decades.

In their books *The Spirit Level* and *The Inner Level*, Richard Wilkinson and Kate Pickett meticulously make the argument, based on hundreds of studies, that the true culprit isn't poverty—it's inequality. Simply put, "People in societies with bigger income gaps between rich and poor are much more likely to suffer from a wide range of health and social problems than those living in more equal societies."[13]

Countries where wealth is distributed more evenly have longer life expectancies and lower rates of health and social problems like mental illness, substance abuse, chronic disease, incarceration, violence, and infant mortality. The issue is not just that more unequal societies have a higher population of poor people inordinately affected by these ills.

Studies show that although these problems are more heavily concentrated among the poor, they are found at higher rates in all socioeconomic levels in unequal societies. The stress of living in a starkly divided community affects everyone up and down the ladder and results in everything from increased rates of violence, to higher levels of stress and depression, to a diversion of resources away from social programs to law enforcement and military.

The United States is the most unequal of all rich countries. In study after study, levels of happiness and life expectancies are lower; infant and maternal mortality rates are higher; rates of mental illness, violence, suicides, and homicides are higher; and more of the population is incarcerated than in countries with smaller socioeconomic divides. These discrepancies can even been seen within countries—between different US states, for example. Those with more equal distributions of wealth and income also have more social support programs and, by almost every measure, a healthier population. Economic inequality and poverty are not random or happenstance occurrences. They result from policies that reinforce hierarchies built on racism, patriarchy, wealth inequities, and other injustices.

Hierarchies, Racism, and Health

Almost all animal groups, including humans, have hierarchical structures. Hierarchies become more problematic when they create steep barriers to rights, resources, and opportunities necessary to survive and thrive for those in the lower ranks. In modern capitalistic societies, your place on the ladder can determine your worth as a human, your access to the prerequisites for health and happiness, your level of exposure to trauma, and the amount of psychological stress you'll have to bear.

Extreme versions of hierarchy found modern societies with European roots can be partially traced back to Descartes and his fellow Western philosophers who confidently decided to put white men like themselves at the top of the pyramid. They alone had fully realized souls, intellectual and emotional capacity, and the ability to feel pain and pleasure. Slightly below the white men were white European women, who also had souls but of a lower quality, and lacked the intellectual capacity of the men. Far below Europeans came the rest of the world, with Africans and Indigenous people at the bottom. These "savages" and "primitives" were not considered fully evolved and had more in common with animals than with white European men. They lacked souls completely and could not feel real emotion or pain, thereby justifying slavery and the colonial project. As Isabel Wilkerson so clearly explains in her book *Caste*, the ranks assigned according to skin tones, gender, ethnicity, and class still persist today. We live in a caste society.[14]

Differences in caste translate into differentials in access to everything from education to housing to food, not because there's a difference in ability or biology between different groups, but because long-held discriminatory beliefs are reflected in societal attitudes, laws, and policies. The result is a stratification of socioeconomic levels within society that mirrors the ranks assigned to different groups, with the lower-caste populations on average at the bottom of the economic ladder. Even apart from socioeconomic differences, membership in a lower caste group is associated with overall higher levels of stress and rates of disease and lower life expectancies. The ongoing effects of racism on the health status of Black, Indigenous, and other people of color is a prime example.

Even though the United States has long-established laws abolishing slavery, Jim Crow–era disenfranchisement, and segregation, the pernicious combined effects of institutional racism and individually held prejudices stubbornly persist. Racial and ethnic minority groups experience higher rates of diabetes, hypertension, obesity, asthma, heart disease, and infant and maternal mortality compared to white populations overall, regardless of socioeconomic status. Most recently, the COVID-19 pandemic has disproportionately affected communities of color with higher numbers of cases, hospitalizations, and deaths than the white populations.

Social isolation and racism are interconnected, and both can be deadly. Harvard professor of public health David R. Williams, one of the preeminent scholars on the complex ways racial discrimination affects physical and mental health, developed scales to measure individual experiences of racism and discrimination. From a very young age, people who experience more prejudice have higher levels of stress hormones and accordingly higher blood pressures and rates of obesity. Experiences of racism can operate similarly to experiences of loneliness and disconnection, leading to stress, inflammation, and further social isolation. People of color must contend not only with prejudice and discrimination on a personal level but also with institutional racism. The healthcare system itself is a prime example of how discrimination is baked into societal structures. Nonwhite racial groups have less access to healthcare, and they receive fewer preventive services and more delayed diagnoses of disease, all exacerbating health disparities.

The legacy of racial segregation shows how difficult it is to effect social change when patterns are so entrenched. Although the Civil Rights Act of 1964 prohibited segregation in public places and businesses, and the Fair Housing Act of 1968 outlawed housing discriminations, maps of urban areas show that segregation persists to this day. Black populations are more likely to be concentrated in areas of higher poverty, worse housing quality, and fewer social resources, like schools, public transportation, grocery stores, hospitals, and medical clinics. Once the caste system is firmly established, it is difficult to eradicate, and the effects reverberate for generations.

Inheritance of Injustice

The United States is built on twin acts of mass trauma inflicted by European colonizers on populations of people deemed at the time to be more like animals than humans. The lasting effects of both the enslavement of Black Africans and the genocide of Indigenous peoples are still with us, causing harm to descendants and damaging communities. The term *historical trauma* refers to the ways subsequent generations feel the effects of violence and oppression perpetrated on their ancestors.

Scholars have studied the effects of historical trauma in families of Holocaust survivors, Native Americans, and African Americans. The mechanism starts with a dominant culture perpetrating mass trauma on a minority population. The victimized group then suffers direct effects manifested in biological, societal, and psychological symptoms. In time, families, communities, and cultural traditions are disrupted and destroyed. Trauma and grief are passed on to subsequent generations in many ways. Descendants inherit a degraded social and cultural environment, as seen in the legacy of racial segregation and the dispossession of the homelands of Native people. Parents transmit the effects of trauma to their children through both emotional and biological pathways. The trauma inflicted on parents and caregivers causes PTSD, high rates of substance abuse, depression, and suicide, affecting how they raise children. Children see and identify with their parents' suffering and experience vicarious trauma.

Trauma is also passed through biological mechanisms. Some of an infant's ability to regulate stress responses throughout life is determined in utero. If a pregnant person has high levels of cortisol, either due to a lifetime burden of stress or adverse experiences during pregnancy, their offspring are more likely to be highly sensitive to stress and to struggle with depression and anxiety later in life.[15]

In recent years evidence has emerged that historical trauma can even alter the expression of the genome in subsequent generations. The new field, called epigenetics, studies how genes are turned on or off and the ways these alterations can be passed down through generations. One of the earliest studies found that Dutch women who experienced famine during World War II passed on a genetic marker that led to worse health outcomes for their offspring. Those children who were in utero during the famine had an increased risk of obesity, high cholesterol, diabetes, and even schizophrenia later in life.[16] In their book *Inflamed: Deep Medicine and the Anatomy of Injustice*,

Rupa Marya and Raj Patel make the important point that although the genetic effect of historical trauma is a biological process, it is a societally determined one. "Epigenetic markers are signs of deeper disease—the social, economic, political and ecological conditions that manufacture trauma, which is passed on, generation after generation."[17] Supporting individuals and communities in overcoming personal and generational histories of trauma is essential, but we must also ask how we can break the cycle and build communities of care that serve as centers of resilience and healing. Part of the answer must be accountability and taking responsibility for past harms and injustices, including reparations.

Ubuntu

Throughout my life, I've been lucky to live in many tight-knit and supportive communities. As a result of seeing my Italian grandparents' generosity and many close relationships in their working-class Buffalo neighborhood, I might have picked up both a craving for connection and also some examples about how to build community. I've become a student of what makes a healthy community, the ways community can be fostered and encouraged, and how we might prevent forces that tear communities apart. Among my teachers have been my chosen family of radical activists in southern Chile, my former neighbors on the Near West Side of Cleveland, and my coworkers and friends in rural Mozambique. If we care to seek them out and listen, there are lessons to be learned from cultures and communities all over the world about how to promote and protect social cohesion and resist the forces of racism and discrimination.

In 1993 I had the opportunity to spend a year of medical school in Chile. I joined a class of students at the University of Concepcion who had started their studies under the Pinochet dictatorship but would finish in a fledgling democracy. I arrived in the country just after a plebiscite ended Augusto Pinochet's presidency in 1988 with the famous "no" vote, although he would continue as commander-in-chief of the Chilean Army for another ten years. My friends included recently returned exiles and activists who had stayed in the country and endured imprisonment and even torture. A Chilean family took me under their wing and taught me meaning of the term *mutual aid*. During the dictatorship, when a neighbor in their town on the outskirts of Concepcion was imprisoned or exiled (a common occurrence), friends would come forward to ensure that the spouse and children had housing, clothing, and food. These expressions of solidarity and resilience strengthened community ties and allowed many people to survive the dark years of oppression and state violence.

I experienced another example of intentional community building when I moved back to Ohio after my residency in family medicine to take a job at a community clinic in Cleveland. The Near West Side neighborhood at that time was diverse in racial, ethnic, and socio-economic terms. Eastern European immigrants landed there fleeing poverty and conflict from the late nineteenth century up until the aftermath of World War II. Puerto Ricans and Mexicans had moved in from the 1940s to the 1960s seeking work in the steel mills. Central Americans came fleeing violence in their home countries in the 1980s and 1990s. A smattering of gentrifiers had moved in but mostly confined themselves to one or two streets.

My home was just a block away from the clinic, and my patients were also my neighbors and friends, some of whom had grown up in the neighborhood, but many had moved there intentionally, attracted by a special spirit of solidarity that seemed to infuse the entire community. There were the Corrigans and the Merrimans, who came to practice their deeply held Catholic faith by living in solidarity with the poor. They were our neighborhood elders when I moved in, the anchors who taught all of us by example how to practice radical hospitality. We all got to know and care deeply for each other through frequent multigenerational multiracial potlucks, knitting nights, spontaneous music nights, and free community yoga sessions.

The Catholic Worker house was a touchstone of the neighborhood, as was the radical church headed by a priest who kept safehouses for fleeing Central American refugees. Catholic anarchist and pacifist Dorothy Day founded the Catholic Worker movement as another kind of manifestation of mutual aid in the 1930s. Almost 200 Catholic Worker communities remain, including the hospitality house in Cleveland where volunteers live together with those needing shelter and food. Day believed that "the mystery of poverty is that by sharing in it, making ourselves poor in giving to others, we increase our knowledge and belief in love." Many folks came as Jesuit volunteers or Catholic Workers and then stayed in the neighborhood to raise their families. Although for many people, religion was the root of their commitment to compassion, no one cared what religion you practiced or if you practiced none at all.

The radical notion that resources should be shared infused the neighborhood, be it housing, food, or just a helping hand. Everyone knew, for example, that the Corrigans had a pickup truck that could always be borrowed in a pinch. A friend explained it with a story. She didn't have a car when she first moved to the community and would walk to the supermarket and inevitably buy more than she could carry home on foot. She never worried too much because every time, she met other neighbors at the store who would give her and her groceries a lift home. You don't need a special mutual aid organization when the ethics of compassion, generosity, and shared responsibility are baked into the community.

This idea that people would come together reciprocally to support each other materially in times of injustice and adversity is not new, but its popularity has waned in the United States and elsewhere. The practice is different from charity in that there is a deep recognition that although today I may be the one giving aid, tomorrow I could be the one in need. The COVID-19 pandemic, even as it deepened isolation and divisions in many places, also spurred a resurgence of mutual aid groups across the country.

Many cultures raise the importance of family and community above that of the individual and weave this vital idea of togetherness into the fabric of their societies, so it's the rule rather than the exception.

After I had been in Cleveland for few years, I was offered a job with a nonprofit organization working to scale up HIV treatment in government health clinics in central Mozambique. I lived in the Shona-speaking part of the country that also encompasses eastern Zimbabwe. In the Shona languages, greeting someone you haven't seen in a while goes something like this:

"Hey, Wendy, how are you?"

"Oh! Molly, hello! I'm okay if you're okay. How are you?"

"Well, I'm okay if you and also your family are okay. How is your mom?" (A long discussion then ensues about the status of all close relatives.)

"So, you and your family are all okay? I'm okay too then."

"Yes, and if you and your family are all doing well, I'm feeling good as well."

The greeting takes several minutes, with neither party seeming impatient nor rushed to get to the point. Checking in on each other and all the loved ones *is* the point. The long greeting stems from the philosophy of Ubuntu. Although the word comes from the Zulu language, almost all the Bantu tongues of southern and central Africa have some version of it. The meaning has been described as "the belief in a universal bond of sharing that connects all humanity." In more academic terms, an article in the *African Journal of Social Work* puts it this way:

A collection of values and practices that people of Africa or of African origin view as making people authentic human beings. While the nuances of these values and practices vary across different ethnic groups, they all point to one thing—an authentic individual human being is part of a larger and more significant relational, communal, societal, environmental and spiritual world.[18]

Distilled to its essence, it means: "I am because you are." The individual human, like an individual honeybee, is not a fully meaningful creature when completely divorced from the context and community they are embedded in.

Bridging the Divides

Building and maintaining community connections was a built-in feature of most of our ancestors' cultures. My forebears were mostly farmers who immigrated to the US from Sweden, Germany, and Italy. In my grandmother's hometown in the Italian Alps, the dense village of dwellings and shops is surrounded by open fields where each household cultivates a garden plot. On the edge of the river that runs through the valley below the town, you'll find a shelter and some fish-cleaning stations. In my grandmother's childhood, the mountains surrounding the town were open to everyone for summer grazing of livestock. Having shared resources that everyone helps caretake binds a community together in common cause. I consider myself lucky to live in one of the few US communities that still practices these old traditions. Our community in New Mexico shares the scarce resource of water, and we come together several times a year to caretake our acequia, or irrigation system.

This past year, as usual, I showed up a little late for the ditch cleaning. Early rising has never been my thing. At the appointed meeting spot, I found our mayordomo, Phil Villarreal, still there handing out assignments. He directed to me to the place where I could meet my crew. We were assigned to the stretch of acequia near the old one-room schoolhouse in the valley, now an adobe ruin that has long since been taken over by pack rats and their bat cousins. I drove down the dirt driveway and noted the cars. My neighbor Mike's was there along with a few others I hadn't seen before. One older model Toyota Corolla was adorned with bumper stickers proclaiming "9/11 was an inside job" and "Illegal immigrants are criminals." When I approached the group of my coworkers for the day, I correctly identified the owner of the Toyota by his Infowars baseball cap. Along with him and my neighbor were two young men in their twenties who were hired to help augment the local labor. They spoke mostly Spanish to each other and when I inquired in Spanish where they were from, they said Chihuahua. It promised to be an interesting day.

As we raked the acequia floor and dug out the gopher holes and sustained scratches from the wild rose and buffaloberry thorns, we got to know each other. The Infowars fan was named Alex. He had a tech job he could do remotely and moved to the valley recently from Wisconsin. When I told him I was a doctor, the talk quickly turned to the COVID vaccines, which he had not gotten and didn't intend to get. Woven in between the small talk was the necessary communication to complete day's tasks. We discussed how deep we should dig out the dirt that had accumulated in the bottom of the ditch from leaf humus and the piles left by the gophers, how aggressive we should be in cutting back the overgrown brush, how far away we should throw the raked leaves so they wouldn't fall back into the ditch with the next rain, and when the work looked finished enough to move on to the next section. There were five of us, Alex, Mike, Jesus, Eugenio, and me. We were a well-oiled machine. Working on a shared project brings people together. We were all able to connect and cooperate in working toward our common goal, and even when the conversation turned to vaccines or theories about origins of the pandemic, it was respectful. No one changed their mind, we just focused on what unites rather than what divides and realized that our common dependence on the land was more important than anything else. Later, in the slanted afternoon sun, all of us sore and scuffed up, we admired our work and imagined the strong stream of water that would soon flow unencumbered through the valley to fill the waiting ditch and flood our gardens and orchards.

Those of us who share the responsibility to maintain our irrigation system in my village are called parciantes, an archaic Spanish word that refers to the portion of the water that each family had the right to use. The emphasis historically was on the common resource that all had to maintain and equitably partition. Our acequia system dates from the late nineteenth century when the communities of Chupadero and Rio en Medio in the next valley over came together to build a diversion high in the mountains so that both valleys could maximize the spring runoff for their crops and pastures. For generations, agreements that governed the acequia systems in New Mexico were more likely to be oral than written, handed down from elders to younger descendants. When disputes inevitably arose, they were handled by the community informally and personally. Although in our modern times, the acequias are governed by written laws and regulations, the water associations that oversee the maintenance of the ditches and the distribution of water still manage to handle most conflicts internally. The fundamental building block of the entire system is trust, a trust built over time and experience. While in many communities the trust that binds together the social fabric has become hopelessly frayed, in Chupadero we constantly work to maintain the threads that tie us to one another. Coming together to repair and restore our common resource builds our relationships with our neighbors and spills over into other kinds of collaborations and gatherings.

Systemic Solutions

As a doctor, I see every day how important social connections are to my patients. Those who have strong ties to family or a close network of friends are far more likely to overcome their health challenges, from chronic illness to addiction to depression and anxiety. Over time and many visits, I'm able to learn more about my patients' lives, but our healthcare system does not facilitate that kind of relationship building. In medical school and residency, I was taught that I should take a complete history and physical on each patient—including asking detailed questions about their medical history and their social environment. In reality, I rarely saw this practice modeled during my training. Our profit-driven healthcare system demands that we see twenty or more patients a day, spending only a few minutes with each. There is little time or space for activities that can't be coded and billed. By default, we learn to focus almost exclusively on the physical symptoms that our education has thoroughly prepared us to address. We shy away from the murky waters of talking about the emotional pain patients experience. That's the province of behavioral health practitioners. At best, we might use a standardized screening tool to diagnose depression and then refer to a therapist or prescribe antidepressants. We just don't have the time or training to diagnose or treat loneliness and disconnection. Even if we do carve out time to discuss emotional and social problems, our solutions are mostly focused on individual behaviors, suggesting ways patients can take the initiative to connect with others. Just like our advice to patients who are overweight, our prescriptions end up asking the individual to take responsibility for fixing what is mostly a social problem. We have even less time or training to address real societal roots of racism, inequality, and disconnection.

Expecting healthcare workers to participate in community transformation may seem radical, but it's one "treatment" that will have lasting results. In his book *How to Be an Anti-Racist*, Ibram X. Kendi suggests that "the only way to undo racism is to consistently identify and describe it—and then dismantle it." That prescription applies not only to our healthcare system but to our society at large. The task seems overwhelming, where to start? Clarissa Pinkola Estés suggests beginning with what is right in front of you. She writes, "Ours is not the task of fixing the entire world all at once, but of stretching out to mend the part of the world that is within our reach. Any small, calm thing that one soul can do to help another soul, to assist some portion of this poor suffering world, will help immensely."[19] We don't have to feel alone and overwhelmed with the task; examples abound of how to bring the philosophy of Ubuntu into our daily lives if we are open to them.

Look around your own community and you will undoubtedly find places where you can practice challenging your own biases and connecting with others who may be outside your normal social sphere—places like libraries or community gardens or neighborhood clubs. Sociologist Ray Oldenburg calls these "third spaces," where people can socially interact with little pressure. These spots might look like coffee shops, dog parks, or community centers. They still exist, although they're becoming more and more endangered; and there's some evidence that they can help combat loneliness and foster a greater sense of well-being.

If you want to go further, reach out to individuals who might be outside your comfort zone, or about whom you have stereotypical ideas. Communicate thoughtfully, with humility and the intent to simply listen, learn, and empathize—while respecting personal boundaries. As with my conspiracy-theory-believing neighbor, you might be surprised at the common ground you find. Take the example of Daryl Davis, a Black musician who started a side gig befriending card-carrying members of the Ku Klux Klan. Through his personal connections and genuine relationships, he has convinced over 200 to give up their robes (which he collects). Davies says the key is genuine interest and curiosity about the other. "If you spend five minutes with your worst enemy—it doesn't have to be about race, it could be about anything . . . you will find that you both have something in common. As you build upon those commonalities, you're forming a relationship and as you build about that relationship, you're forming a friendship. That's what would happen. I didn't convert anybody. They saw the light and converted themselves."[20]

Almost all the regrets of my patients who are dying have to do with the quality of their relationships. Either not being present enough to their family, not keeping up with friends, or not mending fences with people they became estranged from. Being close to death seems to sharpen our sense of what's truly important in life. How might we cultivate that sense of the importance of our connection to others in the rest of our lives, long before those last moments?

9

Embracing Death

Perhaps the easiest way of making a town's acquaintance is to ascertain
how the people in it work, how they love, and how they die.

—ALBERT CAMUS, *THE PLAGUE*

Thwap. The sound reverberated throughout the house, coming from
the French windows near the birdfeeders. As I jumped up from the
couch, I knew what I would find. A young flicker was lying on the red
concrete patio next to the front door, twitching in the final moments
of her life. I cradled the still-warm body, a handful of feathers lighter
than air. A long tongue protruded from her slack, open beak, her black
eyes still suggested a twinkle of life, but her head flopped to one side as
if attached to the body by only a thread, not by bone and sinew. Just
the day before I'd watched that same almost-grown adolescent hop
around the yard after her parents, begging to be fed even though she
seemed perfectly capable of feeding herself.

I wondered if flickers have funeral rituals like magpies do. When
one of their own has passed, magpies fly off to find offerings for the
deceased and swaddle the body in a bed of grasses and plants. They
surround their fallen friend, caw loudly, and gently nudge and preen
the corpse. Other magpies hear the call and come to join the ritual. As

many as forty have been seen in loud raucous displays of grief that can last minutes or hours.[1] One spring, I witnessed an epic magpie/raven conflict. A group of much larger ravens had destroyed a carefully constructed dome of sticks encasing a magpie home and a few new hatchlings—a raven delicacy. Although the magpies called on all their kin to join the battle, there was nothing they could do to dissuade the ravens from their objective. After the loud ruckus died down, one lone magpie remained for several hours perched on the top of the big juniper that contained the ruined nest. She repeated a soft, mournful call I had never heard from the magpies before.

For years it was considered sacrilegious in scientific circles to claim that animals might have emotions like grief, but how else to explain these magpie rituals, or the funerals of elephants or chimpanzees? How else are we to explain the behavior of the orca named Tahlequah, who supported her dead calf for seventeen days, swimming over 1,000 miles before finally letting go and watching the small body drift down to the bottom of the sea? Many animals allow space and time for their grief or perform rituals to mark a passing, but increasingly humans do not.

Even before the COVID-19 epidemic took away our last good-byes for a time, death and grieving had become marginalized, medicalized, and diminished. Most of us will die in a hospital, some number in the ICU or emergency room, with tubes stuck down our throats and in our veins, often surrounded by strangers trying to save us from the inevitable, no matter the cost, rather than our loved ones giving us sustenance for our journey to the other side.

In the United States, grief is subjected to clinical limits. The ICD-10 manual of medical diagnoses permits six months of grief before it is classified as pathological. As many of 60 percent of us will meet the DSM-5 criteria for major depression sometime during the first year after the death of a loved one. How can something be pathological if the majority of us experience it? Rather than give space and support for sadness at the loss loved ones, no matter how long it lasts, we allow just few days or weeks for mourning then the message is: "buck up," or at least have the decency to hide your grief away from others in polite society. If you can't comply, your doctor will likely suggest that you medicate your sadness away.

Medicalized Death

When I started medical school in the autumn of 1990, the first classroom I entered before any other coursework or clinical experiences was the gross anatomy lab. My group of five eager young students spent four hours every day with our assigned cadaver. I'm not certain how the tradition of kicking off medical school with the dissection of the human body began. My lab-mates and I speculated it was to weed out the weak-stomached, or maybe to desensitize us to clinically touching and cutting the human body. Perhaps it was to inure us to the idea of death.

Most of us had never seen a dead body like this before, stripped naked and simply embalmed with none of the tricks that morticians use to make our deceased loved ones appear like they are comfortably sleeping, swathed in the silk linings of their coffins.

Since Tolstoy wrote *The Death of Ivan Ilyich*, not much has changed about how the healthcare system treats death. The medicalization of death, the isolation of the dying, and the ostracization of those grieving are now prevalent phenomenon throughout Western cultures.

As doctors, we are subtly taught to discriminate between the dying person and their affliction. Our training focuses almost exclusively on the disease, the function, the technical process. Since we do not learn much about the dying person's experience of death, we implicitly conclude that it's unimportant—not in our repertoire, more the purview of hospice nurses and social workers and other so-called ancillary staff.

In my first few months as a family medicine intern at the University of New Mexico, I was given the task of talking with an extended family from the Navajo Nation about their relative on my team's ICU service. The patient was in a coma and there was little hope for survival; she was essentially brain dead. I was asked to explain the situation to the family and to answer their questions, alone, without any support from my teachers. The mundane busy work relegated to interns that no one else wants to do is often called "scut work." Did the team consider this duty so unimportant that they thought a new intern could do it unsupervised? A mantra in fast-paced medical education is "See one, do one, teach one." I had never seen anyone break the news to a family of their elder loved one's imminent death.

Before I entered the ICU family waiting room, my chief resident counseled me to be careful talking to the family. He explained that it's considered a cultural faux pas to talk about the death of a loved one or even say the word—it's as if you are wishing them dead. With this one-minute anthropology lesson, I was pushed off to complete my task. I walked with trepidation to the cramped, dimly lit family waiting room across from the ICU. As I opened the door, I saw the large Diné family standing shoulder to shoulder, some of the older ones seated, given places of honor on the two overstuffed chairs and the shabby sofa. I wondered how I was going to explain to them their grandmother was going to die without naming it.

I had heard about Diné end-of-life customs, that those who are dying are expected to leave the family compound and die outside, alone, far away from the rest of the community. I had been told that Navajos fear being around a dead body, so there is no formal funeral as we have in Western culture. Many of my white colleagues shook their heads at the cruelty of these practices when describing them to me. It all seemed consistent with my chief resident's hasty advice. Years later I learned that Navajo rituals had changed dramatically in the 1600s when the Spaniards arrived, bringing with them diseases that would wipe out over 80 percent of the Indigenous population. The Diné quickly observed that those who cared for dying relatives and those who prepared the body often became ill themselves and died shortly after. From this experience, the tradition developed of dying alone, apart from the community. The deceased's possessions were burned, the place where they died was "quarantined" if it was inside a shelter, and the funeral ceremony minimized contact with the body. In other words, the death rituals of the Diné were acts of survival and sacrifice, an intelligent adaptation to the challenges their society faced, and a poignant expression of care for the whole community in time of crisis and genocide.[2]

I took a deep breath and entered the room. In front of me were ten or fifteen relatives of the woman I had previously seen only as a patient, lying prone and lifeless in the hospital bed, her face obscured by the ventilator mask, her eyes taped shut to prevent them opening and drying out, her small, frail form surrounded by a nest of tubing and a collection of humming and beeping machines. In their eyes and faces, I saw reflected the importance and meaning her life held for the family. We were all pressed together in the windowless room as I paused to gather my thoughts. I explained as well as I could that their grandmother was already gone, that there was no hope of recovery. The family sighed and nodded; they were not surprised by the news. We sat together in silence for a while. I wondered if I had offended them. The woman's son asked me a few questions about what would happen next, and then they all thanked me for coming to talk to them, for spending time. They said no one had done that in the week they had been at the hospital. We are trained in medicine about treatments, cures, interventions, solutions. We are taught almost nothing about what to do when there is no cure.

Death Deniers

Since 2020, grief seems ever-present. Some days I think I can almost see it, like a thick tropical mist hanging in the air. Each day brings new reasons to grieve. Black men and women murdered at the hands of cops, grandmothers perishing from COVID-19, countless trees and wildlife extinguished by fires, tens of thousands of innocent people dying in conflicts from Gaza to Sudan—so much death that the grief is staggering. The overwhelming death and devastation around us leads to a place of denial. It becomes too much to comprehend.

Stalin famously said, "If only one man dies of hunger, that is a tragedy. If millions die, it's just a statistic." In the United States alone, we've lost over one million lives to the coronavirus. During the height of the pandemic, journalists tried to break the numbers down into bite-sized chunks that our minds can digest. They told us it's like a 9/11 every three days, or a jumbo jet crashing each day for two years. Still, those among us who have not personally lost a loved one to the pandemic find comfort in refusing to believe it could happen to us. Because our meager rituals are hidden away, it's easy for those who prefer to ignore the cold reality of death to keep their heads firmly buried in the sand.

The Connection Between Sorrow and Joy

Denying death isn't possible everywhere. When I lived in Mozambique in the early 2000s, my home was on the route from the church to the cemetery. All day every Saturday and Sunday a steady stream of flatbed trucks rumbled by filled with mourners pressed closely together, swaying and embracing and supporting each other. Their wails and songs punctuated my weekend with notes that stretched as they passed, making the tones especially doleful. Mozambicans live in a country with high rates of HIV and infant mortality, so they are well acquainted with death. Almost everyone sees a dead body or experiences the passing of a loved one while they are still in childhood. Death is not hidden away. The rituals around dying and grieving are ever-present and impossible to ignore—even if one doesn't live on the road to the graveyard. While healthy respect and space for grieving are built into the culture, the Mozambicans I encountered also know how feel great joy. Celebrations of birth or marriage can be many-day raucous affairs. I came to understand that the Mozambican embrace of death is directly related to their deeply felt expressions of joy.

In Bhutan, which judges national success on a "gross national happiness" index rather than the more common gross domestic product, there is a cultural expectation to think about death at least five times a day. The president of the Centre for Bhutan Studies and Gross National Happiness Research, Dasho Karma Ura, credits mindfulness practices like meditation and yoga, living close to nature, community cohesiveness, and thinking frequently about death for the fact that Bhutanese are, as a society, happier than their income levels would otherwise predict. Ura told a BBC reporter, "Rich people in the West, they have not touched dead bodies, fresh wounds, rotten things. This is a problem. This is the human condition. We have to be ready for the moment we cease to exist."[3]

Honoring death with communal observances and giving those who are grieving license to feel their sadness completely may be more effective than any antidepressant medication in helping to overcome difficult losses. For a person deep in despair, there is nothing so therapeutic as to feel embraced, supported, and loved by family and community, without any expectation of "snapping out of it" on a predetermined timeline.

Knowing we will be cared for and accepted in our anguish when we lose a loved one is comforting, but living close to death can also make us happier in our day-to-day lives. A slew of research shows that those who are at the end of life, whether they are older or have a terminal illness, are much more likely to focus on relationships of people close to them, and on the present moment, rather than on "bucket list" experiences or ambitious plans for the future. The studies show that this kind of mindfulness and focus on everyday pleasures is related to greater overall happiness. Older people are less burdened by stress, more likely to have positive emotions, and dwell more on good memories while minimizing the bad ones. Developmental psychologist Laura Carstensen, a founding director of the Stanford Center on Longevity and a leading researcher of aging and the perspectives of those close to death, has dubbed this the "socioemotional selectivity theory," the idea that those who are near death often have healthier and happier attitudes about life because they are most focused on the things that give their life true meaning.[4]

A growing death awareness movement encourages us to bring death into our daily lives, not only to normalize thinking and talking about it but also to think about what kind of death we desire. Organizations like Death over Dinner and the End Well Project prod us to learn what we can expect at the end our lives and talk about how we might take control of the decisions that are often left to flummoxed and distressed loved ones. New ways of dealing with the end of life involve hospice and palliative care and the assistance of death doulas to help ease our passage. Although these services can provide critical support for families, they also allow us to outsource intimate care and connection with our dying loved ones. We may all want, and even plan for a "good" death, but statistically, few of us will get it. Currently only 25 percent of us die at home. We spend an average of $80,000 on healthcare in our last year of life, often trying to forestall the inevitable end at any cost without fully understanding the consequences. Individual planning can only go so far when, as a culture, we remain invested in pushing death to the margins and banishing it to hospitals and nursing homes.

Some people have taken the popular urge to deny the reality of our final passing to extremes, thinking they can actually outsmart death. Over the past two decades, centers for longevity research have become the new hot trend in academic medicine, spawning a "longevity industry" with attendant startups, major conferences, professional associations, and eager investors. Fringe researchers are supported by those rich enough to think that they can buy immortality like any other commodity. They are looking for the ultimate "biohack" that might allow sufficiently rich humans to extend their healthy lifespan by decades or even centuries. They believe they can make the end of life "optional," at least for those with enough money to buy the cure for death. After millions of dollars spent on supplements and procedures like injecting the plasma of young people, spending time in hyperbaric chambers, and subjecting the body to ultra-cold temperatures, no remedies to mitigate aging have emerged as powerful and simple as the tried-and-true recommendations: daily exercise, good diet, and close friends and family.

The Ordinary Instant

My father never had time to plan his death because he and my mom were too busy planning their semi-retirement years. They had just started thinking of buying an RV, since road trips exploring backroads were among their favorite pastimes. Every summer Dad and Mom would take a few weeks off to drive across the country to visit me. They'd stay with me only for a couple of days. I think I was just the excuse they needed to wander for a few weeks. One late summer, they embarked on one of their more ambitious trips. The plan was to drive the edges of the country from their home in Columbia, South Carolina, to Seattle, where I was living at the time. Their rambling route started on I-10, along the Gulf Coast, then dove down to the Rio Grande, following it to Big Bend National Park, where they stayed in the park's lodge. In the morning, they ate breakfast and went on a short hike. About an hour into the walk, my famously stoic father complained of feeling a weird pressure in his shoulders. They cut the hike short and went back to the room. After a rest and some water, the pressure went away, but they agreed to be safe and call an ambulance to take him to the nearest hospital, about two hours away. Dad was already feeling better and when the ambulance finally arrived, it all seemed like overkill. Mom said, "See you in a bit," as the paramedics wheeled him away. She went back to pack the room up and then followed in the car to the hospital. As she rounded the last curve before exiting the park, she saw the ambulance parked in a turnout on the side of the road and immediately felt a sense of doom. Dad's heart had stopped and he couldn't be resuscitated.

In her book about her husband's death, *The Year of Magical Thinking*, Joan Didion writes that "life changes in an instant, an ordinary instant."[5] My father used to joke that he wanted to die suddenly, musing that getting hit by a bus would be nice. He didn't get the bus, but he got the rest of his wish, in a beautiful, sacred place rather than the hospital-bed death that he dreaded. For my mother, it was the life-changing ordinary instant.

Years ago, I decided that on the tenth year anniversary of Dad's death I'd go to Big Bend and place some kind of secret descanso memorial to him in the spot where he died. *Descanso* is the term given by the Spanish to roadside shrines that commemorate people who died in car accidents. The word means "rest," and traditionally it's where the pallbearers rested on their walk to the cemetery.

I bought a small travel camper so I could be safe traveling in the time of COVID-19, but felt guilty about having a luxury my parents had never attained. I drove first to Mom's house in South Carolina. She contributed some things to the box I would bury at the descanso—a bolo tie he wore during their square-dancing stint, a library card he had signed sporting a sticker with his golf handicap on the back, an excellence award pin from his workplace, a Howard Dean for President button. I added a tire pressure gauge he had given me, a ball-marker from the Masters golf tournament, and his last pair of eyeglasses.

As I traveled through the Deep South, making my way from Mom's house to Big Bend, I unwittingly retraced their path. Later I learned that he'd made the same choices I had, leaving the interstate to travel the backroads, dipping down to visit Del Rio on the Mexican border, taking the longer scenic route. I gazed out at the dramatic mountains and desert as I entered the park, thinking of him taking in the same scenery on the last few miles of his final road trip.

In the morning, after setting up camp nearby, I drove up to the lodge where my parents had spent their last night together, then retraced the ambulance's route to the pullout along the road where they had stopped to try to resuscitate my father.

As I drove, I recalled my mother's recounting of those last moments she shared in this world with her husband. She left the lodge about fifteen minutes after the ambulance, and as she was coming around a bend, she felt suddenly chilled and then saw a brilliant blue bird fly in front of the car. She came around the curve and was puzzled to see the ambulance pulled off on the side of the road, and then she knew. She felt it before they told her. It was a full moon the night he died, and my mother said she couldn't look at the moon for months after.

I came around the same bend and pulled into the spot where my father left the earth. It's a gorgeous place, with expansive desert skies and a panoramic view of the craggy Chisos Mountains. I walked off the pavement down an incline to the shade of an enormous prickly pear cactus and dug a shallow hole for the box containing things that still felt like they contained some part of my father. I added a note to him, covered it up, and marked the spot with a heart-shaped ring of stones.

My journey to my father's death place a decade after he died was part of my own special ceremony to commemorate his life and ensure he was remembered and honored. It was also a way for me to meditate on impermanence and on the importance of cherishing what we have before it passes from this realm. A society that no longer has time for these rituals and that hides death away cannot adequately appreciate the preciousness of life.

A Taste of Death

I almost had my own ordinary instant more than a decade ago in Mozambique. I was flying home from a conference in Durban. We had reached cruising altitude in the small turboprop and I had just settled in with a book. Suddenly, there was a loud *bang* and then silence. Silence is not a welcome sound in a turboprop. The plane lilted and drifted a little, like a paper airplane at the top of its arc, and then went into a spiraling nosedive. The other passengers and I waited, holding our breath, thinking we'd come out of it. The seconds passed in slow motion. The ground could not be too far below and soon we'd come crashing into it. I realized without a shadow of doubt in my mind that I was about to die. I reached for my purse on the empty seat next to me so I could clutch it to me and be identified. I wondered if I had time to write "I love you" to my parents. I heard the flight attendant softly moan, but otherwise we were all silent, contemplating our final moments. I tried to pull my purse toward me but could not move my arm. We were coming out of the dive, and the G forces pushed us all back into our seats. As we returned to cruising altitude, the pilot matter-of-factly reported that we would be going back to the Durban airport, as if nothing had happened. I broke into a cold sweat and started vomiting with the intense parasympathetic release that followed the adrenalin surge of coming within a hair's breadth of the end of my life. I thought of my long-dead grandmother and felt her presence with me and somehow wondered if she had been my guardian angel. The next day, a South African newspaper reported that we had pulled out just 700 feet from the ground, the height of a tall skyscraper. The last lines of the article noted that "an American doctor who is working in Mozambique was so shaken she had to be taken from the plane in a wheelchair."

For days afterward, the air seemed to sizzle and each moment had new meaning. My senses were heightened, food tasted better, the feeling of wind on my skin felt like a crisp, tingling embrace. I had shaken hands with death, and now life seemed all the more luscious. I felt somehow chosen, like perhaps I was saved for a reason, and became aware of a strange new imperative to make sure I wasn't squandering my gift of life. The effect lasted only a few weeks, but I sometimes still reflect on the moment and wish I could have bottled that feeling to imbibe later.

Not all of us will have a near-death experience, but all of us can get acquainted with death and come to terms with its inevitability. In doing so, we might better savor and appreciate the miracle of our existence. By integrating this passage into our culture in a more meaningful way, we can not only make our own fragile lives more meaningful, but we can also honor more deeply those who have gone before us.

Honoring Elders

Yet another casualty of pushing death and grieving to the margins of our society is the collective knowledge of our elders. In many Indigenous cultures the experience of death isn't individual or even familial—it's communal. Death is not seen as a final termination but more as a transition. The stories and memories of elders are carefully preserved, living on for generations. As we lose the ceremonies and customs that honor those who have passed, we also lose the parts of our own history contained in them, all contributing to our collective forgetting.

Many cultures have practices of remembrance, like the Day of the Dead, which originated with Indigenous cultures of Mexico, was adopted by the Spanish, and then melded into the particular version of Mexican Catholicism. In all of these ceremonies, those who have passed are honored by retelling their stories and recounting their memories. In this way, death is not final, the elders are remembered, and their sacred stories are passed on.

One lost human memory among many we should be mourning is the experience of an abundant natural world. The earth we have inherited from our ancestors is now nearly devoid of wild places, with only a smattering of the rich biodiversity that our grandparents and great-grandparents knew. For younger generations, our natural areas may seem to be "normal" and "full" of wildlife as they have no context or mental image of the previous richness. The shifting baseline phenomenon occurs when the most recent generation accepts the decimated world as the new standard.

Some observant elders among us have seen and noted the rapid, exponential decline of wild species and ecosystem functioning over the past fifty years. Soundscape recording artist Bernie Krause had no idea he would be documenting the demise of an ecosystem when he started recording the chorus of bird and wildlife sounds thirty years ago near his home, in a state park outside San Francisco. Every April he would return to the same spot near a woodland stream and an enormous maple that itself was an elder in the forest. The recordings helped soothe his ADHD in a way that no medication could. "The only thing that relieved the anxiety was being out there and just listening to the soundscapes," he told a reporter. By the 2010s, when California was in the midst of the worst drought in a millennium, Krause noticed the sounds were drastically diminishing. By April 2023, after drought and successive wildfires dried up the stream and burned down even the ancient maple, his recorder picked up no sounds at all. In his book *The Great Animal Orchestra*, he writes, "A great silence is spreading over the natural world even as the sound of man is becoming deafening. The sense of desolation extends beyond mere silence."[6]

If we don't hear and honor the stories of our grandparents, we will never know what the natural world was like, what was real and possible, just a few decades ago. Without the knowledge of that world, we will inevitably pass down to our children and children's children a sad acceptance of this now-diminished world as the best we can do, without the imagination to fully comprehend what we could aspire to rekindle.

With the loss of cultures and languages through assimilation, oppression, and genocide, we are losing the cultural knowledge our ancestors gleaned though thousands of years, what anthropologist Wade Davis calls the ethnosphere. Each of those cultures found unique ways to answer the question of how we are to live in balance and symbiosis with the natural world. We desperately need the knowledge of all of those elders if we are to overcome the challenges that face us today.

The Death of Nature

In New Mexico during the spring of 2020, thousands of migratory birds fell from the sky, emaciated, dead, or dying from hunger and hypothermia due to an unseasonably early cold snap. There were reports of hundreds of swallows, warblers, bluebirds, sparrows, and blackbirds strewn across the gypsum dunes at White Sands National Park or lethargically struggling on the ground in the forests of northern New Mexico. Ornithologists speculated that the wildfires in California obligated a too-early migration, before the birds had built up enough reserves for their journey, and also forced them into a longer and unfamiliar route over the Rocky Mountains rather than straight down the coast. The cold snap robbed them of insects for a few days, just enough to push them over the edge in their already weakened state. The magnitude of the die-off was called unprecedented, but a similar event happened earlier the same year in Europe when cold weather and strong winds led to the deaths of thousands of swallows crossing over the Mediterranean from Greece to Africa.[7]

Mass die-off events, affecting hundreds of thousands or even millions of animals, are becoming more common; most are attributed to a combination of disease, lack of food, and erratic climate events.[8] Just as we feel the loss of one life more acutely than the numbing deaths of thousands, so too do we mourn the extinction of a single species more deeply than the great "thinning" of wildlife that has marked the last hundred years. In the past century, most of those events have had human fingerprints at the crime scene. Some were unintentional, like the extinction of the passenger pigeon, which had seemed so abundant that wiping them out was inconceivable. Other events were quite deliberate, like the Chinese effort to eradicate sparrows in the 1950s as one of the "four pests" along with rats, mosquitos, and flies. Mao believed that sparrows were eating rice from paddy fields and warehouses, so millions and millions of birds were killed. In reality, the birds feasted mostly on the insects that were much more damaging to the crops. An ecological collapse ensued leading to drastically reduced crop yields and directly contributing to the Great Chinese Famine.[9]

The Living Planet Report 2020 warns us that "nature is unravelling and . . . our planet is flashing red warning signs of vital natural systems failure." The report attributes the decrease of wildlife populations by two-thirds in just the past two generations to human activities like logging, mining, development, and, of course, climate change.[10] The losses loom so large, it's not easy to comprehend them. Focused efforts to save species from extinction garner much more attention than larger-scale changes needed to stem this global tidal wave of devastation. The denial of climate change itself might be related to our inability to comprehend the massive numbers of deaths already incurred as a result of our way of living.

From Pushing Death Away to Holding It Close

News of Jack's death spread quickly through the valley, even though we were all ensconced in our homes and the usual potlucks and informal gatherings were no longer happening by mid-summer of 2020.

Jack was loved by everyone in the valley. Even later in life, when cancer had taken much of his strength, he was known for always contributing to collective work on the acequias, gifting his legendary homemade whiskey, and sharing the wisdom he had acquired from his decades living in the community. Although the coronavirus prevented us from gathering to commemorate his life, a spontaneous show of gratitude sprouted on the chain-link fence in front of his workshop. The signs read "Thank You Jack" and "We Love You," a heartfelt expression of communal grieving. Even at the height of pandemic isolation, we refused to grieve alone. We refused to forget.

Our community's observance of Jack's death contrasted sharply with the experience of many of my patients who lost loved ones during the pandemic. Families felt isolated, as if they had to swallow their grief whole, in isolation. Many were unable to say goodbye, and funeral gatherings were impossible. Author Jamie Anderson writes, "Grief is love with no place to go." That might be true in a society where grief is private and individual, but in cultures where grieving is a communal experience, the burden is shared publicly by all and the love is carried forward in every member of the community as remembrance.

In the Western world, we are expected to bear the anguish of losses alone. The burden of compounded sorrows over the last few years seems overwhelmingly enormous for many of us. How much lighter the load if we were not trying to bear the entire weight ourselves, as individuals? What can we learn from the Bhutanese and the Mozambicans and the hundreds of other cultures across the world that allow adequate space and time to honor and remember the dead and share our grief? What would shift if we invited death into our daily lives? Perhaps we might then appreciate the true value of life—all life—and in doing so, live more joyfully, compassionately, and consciously.

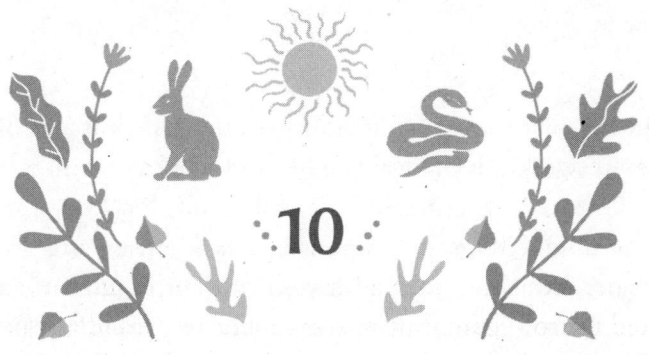

10

Finding Hope

What if it was the people who were regarded by elite Westerners as
brutes and savages—the people who could see signs of vitality, life,
and meaning in beings of many other kinds—who were right all
along? What if the idea that Earth teems with other beings who act,
communicate, tell stories, and make meaning is taken seriously?

—AMITAV GHOSH,
THE NUTMEG'S CURSE: PARABLES FOR A PLANET IN CRISIS

As I approached the farmhouse where I had arranged to stay, I heard
the enthusiastic "Ela mesa!"—an exhortation to "come inside." Ten-
tatively, I entered the family home, took off my shoes, and sat down
at the simple wooden table in the large room that served as kitchen,
dining room, and living room. My hosts—Sofia, Kostas, and their
daughter Maria—set in front of me the customary offering for new
guests and tired travelers, a small dish of sour cherries in light syrup
and a tall glass of cold water. I was instructed to put a spoonful of cherries in the water, or just to eat them right from the spoon. Magically,
I felt the weariness of the past days of planes and taxis and ferries melt

---

* A version of this chapter was previously published in the literary journal *Inkwell*,
Spring 2021.

away. In my first twenty-four hours on the Greek island of Ikaria, I was offered two kinds of local cheese (and met the woman who made them), two kinds of vegetable pie, fish soup, local teas, and several cups of local wine. Figs, pomegranates, blackberries, and grapes grew everywhere. I was told to avail myself of their bounty in addition to taking anything I desired from the vegetable garden just beyond the door of my rental cottage.

As the granddaughter of Italian immigrants and someone who has been welcomed into homes all over the globe, I have learned a few things about hospitality. Among the cultures I have experienced, none can rival Ikaria for its welcoming and generous spirit. After living as an honorary Ikarian for a couple of weeks on the still relatively isolated Greek island in the southeast corner of the Aegean Sea, I glimpsed just how much better life would be if we all could muster that sort of kindness with each other. Just walking by a stranger's home and offering the greeting of "Yassas" will often garner a spontaneous invitation to coffee. During my time there, I hardly spent much on food as I was constantly being fed by friendly grandmothers. I came to this place to see, and viscerally experience, one of the celebrated "Blue Zones," the handful of places on Earth where people seem to live much longer, happier, and healthier lives than the rest of us.

The Blue Zone Phenomenon

The designation of Blue Zones predates by a few years the recent obsession with longevity. The term comes from public health researchers who were studying villages in Sardinia where high numbers of people seemed to be reaching healthy old age, into their 90s and 100s.[1] They drew blue circles around the villages with the longest living inhabitants and noticed a pattern. Later, Dan Buettner, an enterprising journalist and *National Geographic* fellow, joined the Sardinia study epidemiologists to identify four more Blue Zones—in Ikaria, Okinawa, Costa Rica, and among Seventh-Day Adventists in Loma Linda, California.

In the past decade since Buettner published his first article about the phenomenon, trademarked the name, and launched his Blue Zone Project, longevity research has become the next big thing. The search for the fountain of youth now fuels a multimillion-dollar industry as scientists and entrepreneurs search for the holy grail: the specific mix of diet, supplements, exercise, and individual practices that will confer near-immortality—or at least a healthy lifespan well past 100 years. Nascent research is gobbled up by tech CEOs and startups looking to capitalize on the next fad treatment. Already the wealthy seekers practice near-starvation diets, inject the blood of young people into their veins, and spend time in hyperbaric oxygen chambers, all based on scant evidence. Big Medicine has gotten into the game as well. The US National Academy of Medicine recently launched the Healthy Longevity Global Grand Challenge, with a prize of $25 million, and several academic centers have started multimillion-dollar institutes to research the keys to long and healthy lives. They've coined a new moniker for themselves, biohackers, based on the belief that the key to immortality lies merely in cracking the biological code that leads to aging and death.

Daughter of Fortune: An Ikarian Point of View

Maria Katinos grimaces when I mention that I'm traveling to Ikaria because of the Blue Zone designation. She's a daughter of the island. Both her mother and father were born and raised and still live part-time there. Ikaria is in her blood, she says, and she comes back as often as her job in Athens will allow. We meet on the ferry, on our way to her family's homestead. The cottage I'm renting was once a stable for their goats, now renovated for tourists.

Her disdain is understandable. She comes to the island to reconnect with family and friends, to dance, to swim in the pristine sea off secluded rocky beaches, and to escape the stress of her Athens life. To relax—chalará, as the Greeks say—which might be Ikaria's informal motto. She believes that all the focus on longevity misses what's truly special about the place. The gift of a long life has largely bypassed her own family. Two grandparents died in their early seventies of cancer, and her father, just in his late fifties, has already had a couple of coronary artery catheterizations. I learn this as we are all out on the patio talking about family history. Maria and her father, Kostas, are smoking cigarettes.

Although Ikaria and the other Blue Zone cultures may offer lessons on how to live well throughout a long life, Maria and others I met on the island believe that much of what tourists and researchers take away is missing the point. One of the islanders' main lessons is that longevity is not a competitive sport, despite what the scions of Silicon Valley might think. Rather than individual attributes, the secret of the Blue Zones and other places on Earth where people live full and relatively happy lives despite poverty and hardship likely lies in collective factors: the relationship between the people, their community, and their environment.

The Allure of Ikaria

Ikaria has a strong pull for those who have a connection with the island. There are only about 8,000 full-time residents, but you will find diaspora communities throughout the world. Many former sons and daughters return in the summer, and everyone seems to know everyone else. The island has always been isolated, historically threatened by pirates from the rough part of the Aegean Sea on the north coast, so the oldest villages are hidden in the interior mountains in tight-knit communities. The landscape is stunning—impossibly steep terraces built by hand in ancient times harbor olive trees and grape vines hundreds of years old. The combination of soaring rock-faced mountains, steep gorges, and acres of terraced vineyards and orchards makes the land seem incredibly harsh and astonishingly fertile all at once—and Ikarians are almost always outside enjoying it. You'll find them tending their gardens, swimming at hidden beaches, or on their verandas visiting with neighbors. The two side-by-side outdoor cafés in Vrakades, the first town I visited, overflow with conviviality every night as the whole village gathers to share stories of their day along with copious wine, food, and coffee. Informal meals are shared communally, and often everyone eats from the same plate.

Time on the island seems fluid, and people are never in a rush, always open to whatever possibility may present itself. Famously, no one wears a watch, and clocks are in short supply. "Go with the flow" might be another translation of *chalara*. When you ask people what they are going to do later, you might get a rough plan, but likely with a "maybe" attached. Somehow it all works out—you connect with your friends and everyone has fun.

Unlike flashier and better-known islands like Mikonos, Santorini, or even neighboring Samos, the island never attracted wealthy tourists or yachting types, likely because there are no large marinas, and the nightlife consists mostly of huge community feasts called panigyri and the nightly gatherings at the village coffee shop.

Panigyria and Coming Together

While I was there, I had the opportunity to attend a couple of panigyria in the company of native Ikarians who were gracious enough to try to teach me the island's signature dance. The size and style of these gatherings may vary, but they all follow the same general script. Communities come together for a meal of roasted goat, traditional side dishes, and lots of local wine, almost always watered down to modulate the effects for the long hours to come. Musicians gather and begin playing songs of the Aegean Islands and Asia Minor, including the song most closely associated with Ikaria. People quickly begin to dance, in couples or in large circular chains, depending on the type of song. The dancing and drinking continue through the night, often for more than eight or ten hours.

The strains of the iconic song "Ikariotico" go right to the heart of most Ikarians. Maria shows me the goose bumps on her arm as she hears the opening notes. It's impossible not to smile when you are dancing the Ikariotico, at least after you learn the steps, which everyone here does by the age of ten. Everyone locks arms or holds hands in a huge spiral. Gender, age, provenance, or even dancing ability doesn't matter. Some people believe the dancing induces a kind of ecstasy. After experiencing the infectious joy of community, the exuberance of the lead dancers, and the hypnotic repetition, I can see what they mean. Elders are honored at these intergenerational celebrations. Many seventy- and eighty-year-olds are among the most agile dancers. Even those who are too frail get on the dance floor remain much valued and active members of the community. They are seated in places of honor, and everyone comes to greet them during the evening.

I saw no police and heard no sirens during my two weeks on the island. When I inquired about crime, I was told there was very little, largely because everyone knows each other or is connected by family. There are police on the island, I learned, but was told that their duties are mostly focused on busting people for smoking marijuana in public and helping drunk folks get home. Among the native islanders I met, I hardly heard of a divorce either. When I asked about this, I learned that of course there are "indiscretions," but people seem to get beyond them. Conflicts and betrayals among friends and family exist in Ikaria as everywhere in the world, but generally these are forgiven or overlooked in the interest of maintaining good relationships within the community. When it comes to transgressions, Ikarians seem to be able to let things go and move on with grace.

Every place has a garden, and most have chickens or goats. There are over 20,000 beehives on the island. The first morning duty is tending to the animals and plants. In the apartment where I stayed in Akamatra, I was awakened each morning by the spray of water from the hose and the chickens asking to be fed. My hosts, Popi and Despina, who are in their seventies, were already up and merrily attending their chores. Despina came down before noon every day and offered some of her home cooking or fresh eggs from the hens I watched pecking the ground from my balcony.

Difficult Times: War, Starvation, Diaspora

Life might be long for many Ikarians, but it was also hard, especially during the time that most of the island's centenarians were coming into adulthood and raising families. For much of the twentieth century, there was little electricity, few roads good enough for cars, and scant healthcare. People lived off the land and shared their bounty. Contact with mainland Greece was limited, especially before the 1970s, so a bad harvest was dire for everyone. The German and Italian occupation of the island during World War II was particularly harsh and was combined with a British blockade aimed at the Axis powers. The result was a widespread destruction of farms and homes as the invaders took all the harvests for themselves. It's estimated that nearly 10 percent of the island's 12,000 inhabitants at the time succumbed to starvation.[2]

Thousands of Ikarians were forced to leave the island to escape the crushing poverty during the postwar years, but in recent decades many have returned, like Nikos, whom I met in Akamatra. He's a carpenter who worked for twenty years in Australia before coming home in 1982. Nikos left in the 1960s to make a better life working on ships around the world. He briefly tried living in the United States, in Philly (he chuckles, "I was illegal"), but quickly decided it wasn't for him. Everyone was too focused on making money, he said. He asked me, "How is it now?" I responded, "Much, much worse."

We talked about Ikaria and what makes it so special. People here know you don't need much to be happy, he said. There is almost no abject poverty on the island and no elite wealth either. Everyone has housing and access to food. In contrast to the other Greek islands that attract hordes of yacht-owning Europeans, the only signs of profligate wealth I saw during my time there were a large catamaran briefly docked in Magganitis and a yellow sports car I passed on the road. I surmised the latter was likely a tourist, as the driver did not slow or stop politely on the narrow road as we approached each other, me in my beat-up rental Fiat, as all the other Ikarian drivers kindly did.

When I asked if everyone had electricity, Nikos said yes, everyone in the village except one guy who didn't want it and preferred to live in the old way. People help each other out and there are programs for those who may not have enough to eat, he added.

I learned from Nikos and others that Ikaria is known as the Red Island, another friend calls it the "Cuba of the Aegean." It's been the site of exiles, including over 10,000 communists banished there after the Greek civil war, so traditions of welcoming strangers are old and well established. The exiles included artists and musicians, most notably the cherished composer Theodorakis, who wrote the score for *Zorba the Greek*. Imagine if everyone blacklisted during the McCarthy era in the US were exiled to one beautiful island, then you can get an idea of what this did for Ikaria. People here are still on the far-left spectrum of Greek politics, mostly communist and socialist, and fierce in their beliefs.

Nikos asked me why the people of the US tolerate so much oppression. "Why don't they rise up?"

"I don't know," I sadly responded.

As we toured the new house he built on his ancestral land and he showed off his beautiful carpentry, he gestured to the ancient stone dwelling still standing behind the main house. "That is where I was born." It belonged to his grandfather, who emigrated to the US and never came back. "His bones are still in Ohio," Nikos said wistfully. We talked about how Ikaria is changing with the recent uptick of tourists and the Blue Zone attention. "The life, the life is not a number," he said. "Life is quality." Some people are making a little more money on the tourist trade, but he says, "Then they start to look down on us, and they lose the ethos."

Cooking Up Wellness

George Karimalis and Eleni Karimali have come back to Ikaria as well. They both grew up on the island but left for some years to go to university and work in Athens. Now they live on land that's been in George's family for generations. George is a nutritionist and winemaker, and Eleni is a chef. Together they run a small inn on the vineyard but also travel in the winters to offer cooking and wellness workshops in Europe and the United States. They are passionate about educating the world on the traditional Ikarian way of cooking before it becomes forgotten. On the mantel in their kitchen sits a photo of five generations of Eleni's family. She poses with her daughter, grand-daughter, mother, and grandmother. Her grandmother was one of the celebrated centenarians, reaching 102 years of age, but Eleni tells me that her life was hard and filled with a lot of grief: she lost four of her five children in infancy.

I asked George about the secrets of the Ikarian diet. He listed the important elements: plant-based with occasional meat or fish, nothing fried or grilled; everything organic, local, and seasonal, either grown or foraged; lots of fermented foods, from olives to cheese; lots of olive oil, mostly not heated, on salads and in dips like tzatziki and the local fava; lots of herbs, greens, and legumes; no sugar—the only sweeten-ers are local honey or the "grape molasses" made from reduced grape juice; lots of water and a good amount of local wine. Almost everyone makes wine from their own grapes or olive oil from their own trees or both. Although George and Eleni are great evangelists for the Ikarian lifestyle and their way of preparing and eating food is certainly health-ier than our usual diet, it's difficult to transplant into our fast-paced and work-dominated daily schedules.

The Secret of the Ikarian Way

The key to the Ikarian way of life is not one thing or even a list of things. The whole vibe of the place seeps into your skin from the first moments on the island. I ended up experiencing all the different kinds of Greek love on Ikaria—agape, philia, even eros. It's a sensual place—the feeling of floating on gentle waves in the cerulean Aegean, the sounds of chicken, goats, and wild birds in the morning, the first strains of the Ikariotico, the taste of the fresh, homemade delicacies, the morning scents of sage and the sea, earthiness and freshness. And one is never far from stunning views—rocky crags over impossibly terraced hillsides, and always the backdrop of the serene Aegean Sea.

The Ikarians I met taught me to slow down and fully enjoy these sensations. My first day on the island, Kostas picked some tomatoes for lunch and paused to appreciate the aroma of each one, bringing it to his face and breathing in its essence. When George and Eleni visited me in Santa Fe to offer their cooking and longevity workshop in my home, we went to the farmer's market to prepare. They took in all the new aromas and tastes slowly, sensually. When they were offered some new and novel produce—salsa made from tomatillos, for example—they first inhaled it like a fine wine, then took a small taste to savor it completely.

The Pull of the Western Life

Changing desires of the islanders and encroachment of the outside world are shifting some of the very practices that contributed to the extraordinary rates of longevity. The plant-based, microbial-rich local diet extolled by George and Eleni is being slowly replaced by more meat and imported, processed foods. A farmer I met lamented that he is having an increasingly difficult time selling the meat from his small herd of twenty-five cows at a fair price because of the influx of cheaper European Union beef. Some of the conditions that may have contributed to long lives are not how people want to live today. Few Ikarians want to go back to the days before there were many roads and going to the next village meant hours of walking on steep footpaths, when there was no medical care and no grocery stores, even if some elements of that difficult lifestyle kept the people who survived it healthier. Some even argue that the secret of the Blue Zones is that only the most resilient survived.

But the conveniences of the West come at a price. Quick-to-prepare processed foods are not as healthy. Less reliance on locally grown products will not only hurt farmers but also disconnect younger generations of Ikarians from the land. As more longevity tourists pour into the island

and those profiting off them grow more affluent, economic inequality will grow. As the modern world insinuates itself more and more into the Ikarian way of life, a cautionary tale for the Ikarians might be found in the story of another former Blue Zone, in Okinawa, Japan.

A Cautionary Tale

For decades, despite living in one of the poorest provinces, the Okinawan population had the longest life expectancies in all of Japan, a country where people already live longer than any other on Earth. On average, Okinawans still live much longer than their American counterparts, but in recent years, their advantage over their fellow Japanese citizens has eroded. In the decades since 1990, the rates of heart disease and stroke among Okinawans have increased to match and even surpass Japanese averages.

The declines started in the post–World War II era when Americans were welcomed and seen as liberators after oppressive Japanese rule. Okinawa remained under US control until 1972, and during that span, the US military set up several bases and imported thousands of troops, along with all the trappings of American lifestyle and cuisine.

As a result, thousands of Okinawans were displaced from their land and their traditional way of life. The amount of fat in the Okinawan diet went from 10 percent in 1960 to over 30 percent today. Okinawans now have the highest obesity rates in all of Japan,[3] and not coincidentally, a rising mortality rate among younger adults, as well as falling life expectancies overall.[4] The effects of successive waves of colonization, first from the Japanese and then from Americans, have eroded the very aspects of the Okinawan diet and culture that once created conditions conducive to the long healthy lives of its centenarians.[5]

An Impetuous Quest

Ikaria is named for Icarus, who, according to legend, fell from the sky near the island. Icarus's father made them both a pair of wings from wax and feathers so they might escape imprisonment and fly to freedom. He warned Icarus not to fly too close to the sun, but the impetuous boy could not resist. His wings promptly melted, and he plummeted into the sea. The Icarus metaphor might also be applied to those seeking the coveted fountain of youth in our time.

In recent years, thousands of longevity tourists have made their way to Ikaria to try to discern the secret of the island. The centenarians of the Blue Zones have been sought out and interviewed by journalists and researchers so many times, their responses start to blur together as they are turned into sound bites for travel brochures. Entrepreneurs from other countries are swooping in, hoping to capitalize on the newfound fame of the place. Many Ikarians are rightly becoming wary of all the attention. Like animals in zoos, the version of these cultures neatly packaged for marketing is not the same as the real thing in all its complexity. Most Ikarians understand that when their way of life is reduced to a commodity, they risk losing what made their long healthy lives possible in the first place.

Thousands of cultures on earth, especially non-Western and Indigenous cultures, have answered the central question of "how to live well" in unique ways that we need to hear and learn from if we are to extricate ourselves from our current downward spiral. Most of their stories and lessons are largely unknown, and many of these cultures are on the verge of extinction from increasing westernization, commodification, and outright oppression and genocide.

The lessons these healthy cultures have to teach us can't be boiled down to a few diet and lifestyle tips. If we want to reap the benefits their inhabitants enjoy, we'll have to listen carefully to what they have to tell us, as whole communities as well as individual elders. If we do, we might we learn from these places how to infuse our own cultures and communities with the ethos of kindness, generosity, connection to nature and the land, and time for relaxation and to fully enjoy and appreciate the richness of our environments and relationships.

All the millions in longevity research haven't revealed the secrets that the Ikarians know in their bones: health and wellness are collective attributes and come from our relationships with each other and the natural world. The Ikarians have learned this intuitively, they are born into their way of life. Perhaps we also must live it to understand, to find that the true biohacks are collective measures, not individual interventions. Narcissistic longevity-seekers can't quite see that our fates are interwoven. Even in their yachts and mansions, the stress of living in an unequal and increasingly fragmented world reaches them too. Their long-sought silver bullet to prevent aging might look less like a pill and more like a community where everyone is cared for and connected to each other, where the natural world is cherished and its richness is nurtured.

What if the moguls of the world, instead of chasing the latest medical fads with their millions, would invest in solutions that brought us more economic equality? What if they invested in food systems that ensure we all have access to healthy diets with low impacts on our natural environment? What if they invested in renewable energy that doesn't pollute our air and water? What if they invested in public transportation systems, housing, social programs that ensure everyone is cared for? What if they saw all of this not as a list of fixes, but as building an ecosystem for lifelong wellness? What if they came to realize that only way to sustainably ensure their individual well-being, and that of their families for generations to come, was to provide for those basic needs for everyone? Indeed. What if?

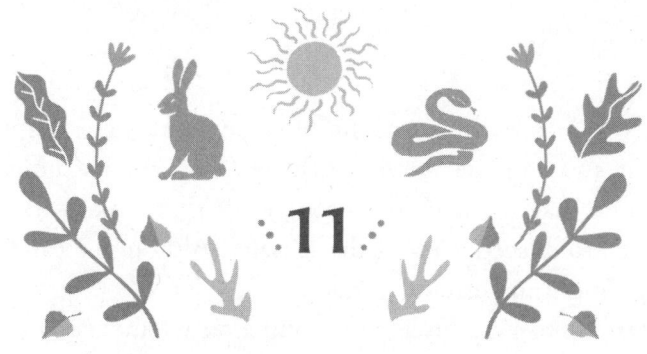

The Path Forward

The time has come for us to reimagine everything. . . . We have to
reimagine revolution and think not only about the changes in our
institutions but the changes we have to make in ourselves.

—GRACE LEE BOGGS

I have a deep friendship with a tree. It stands near the wrought-iron
gate in an adobe wall enclosing the herb garden just outside my back
door. When I first met him, he was a magnificent heart-shaped broadleaf cottonwood. There are many other cottonwoods in the valley, but
most are the narrow leaf variety rather than *Populus deltoides*, the name
given to these plains cottonwoods by European taxonomists for the
triangular shape of their leaves. My friend is one of only two broad-
leafs on the land near my home and the only mature one, probably
around my age, more than fifty years old. The leaves of this particular
species turn a spectacular shade of mango-orange-yellow in the fall.

When I sit on my back porch in the evenings and hear the wind
rustle his leaves, I can imagine I am near an ocean shore listening to
the sound of surf against sand. His branches make a favorite perch
for warblers, a lookout for hummingbirds standing vigil over their
claimed feeders and flowers, and a prime nesting spot for the bushtits'

hanging orb homes. In spring he blossoms with long purple flower stems that sway in the wind. I say "he" because we humans have assigned the male gender to cottonwoods that make catkins rather than the cottony seed pods of the females. Although I can't imagine how trees might understand gender.

He started showing his age not long after we met, as cottonwoods and humans often do after a few score years on this earth. His long, elegant limbs weakened and first one, then another broke off during subsequent windstorms. When the largest branch came down, it cleaved a part of the trunk with it. The morning after this most serious injury, I came out of the house and found him broken, maybe mortally injured, and felt grief-stricken at the thought of watching him wither and die. Hoping to help him live a few more years, I sawed off the branch and tried to repair the rift, bolting the severed part back to the main tree like an arboreal orthopedic surgeon. For a while, his shape was more like a broken heart, a wide V shape. Now, a few years later, branches have sprouted up and filled the void. Growth and healing are possible even after middle age. My friend has a story, and it is intertwined with my story, if I let it be.

This passage might have sounded strange. One does not normally hear the language of relationships between humans applied to non-pet living creatures, especially plants. Some people would call this anthropomorphizing. I am using human concepts, like gender, for my friend because I experience our relationship through my human consciousness. I have no idea what tree consciousness is like or how he "sees" me, but I believe that a kind of tree consciousness exists, even if some botanists would shudder at my use of the word. In recent years, the debate over plant intelligence has intensified, with esteemed biologists coming down on both sides. More and more research shows that plants can communicate with each other. They have memories. They can learn. They exhibit altruism and even recognize their kin.

Suzanne Simard's groundbreaking work on the relationships between "mother trees" and the rest of the forest was denigrated by ecologists for years, but she finally overcame the naysayers with impeccable and irrefutable evidence. She found that parent trees communicate and support their offspring and other vital plants through a mycelial network—tiny threads of fungus that form an intricate web in the soil and pass messages and nutrients back and forth.[1] Other researchers have observed that when an elder tree is injured, or even cut down, the brethren trees around it rally to support her and give her life even if only a stump remains.[2]

Anthropocentrism can blind us to the possibility that other living beings can share our "uniquely" human qualities, like emotion, intelligence, free will, or consciousness. For centuries, humans have made this mistake with other animals. The bright line once imagined between animals and humans is quickly being erased; mounting evidence says that the ability to cooperate and plan, play and express joy, and even have rituals and culture is not unique to our species, or even just to mammals. Some people may bristle reflexively at the thought that plants have a kind of higher intelligence. Consider that any interpretation of the motivations or behaviors of trees or animals is necessarily anthropocentric—filtered through our human minds, which often work in binary, either imagining that all living things experience the world as humans do or completely rejecting that notion. Both assumptions seem arrogant. Maybe the Venn diagram of human and other-than-human experience of the world is neither two concentric circles nor two separate circles. Maybe they overlap in ways not easily comprehended. Science has little tolerance for accepting the mystery of how a tree or an elephant or an octopus understands their existence. Yet we are learning that almost all living things, from plants to insects to fish to mammals, do have a consciousness and methods of communication they use to interpret their world and convey their reality to others.

How else to explain the intricate decision-making process of bees when they are faced with the task of finding a new nest? In his book *Honeybee Democracy*, Thomas Seeley explains that when a honeybee swarm chooses a new nest, the process looks like the collective, consensus decision-making that one might find in a small-town citizens' meeting. When honeybees swarm, they send out scout bees to find another home for their colony. The scouts come back and act like competing candidates, working to convince their sisters that their find is the best possible new dwelling. Unlike opposing political parties, the bees are united in their understanding of what attributes they are seeking. The process is one of storytelling, explanation, debate, and consensus building, all accomplished through waggling movements.[3]

The scout bees return from their search missions and dance expressively in specific circles, jigs, tail shakes, and wing flutters that together describe in detail the positive characteristics of their chosen prospect. They must first convince those immediately around them on the surface of the swarm, and those nearby bees convince others, until the whole hive agrees on the best spot. There is no personal gain for the bee whose discovery is chosen, and in fact, dangerous scout jobs are taken up by elders who have spent most of their life foraging so know the terrain well. When they sense their community needs to swarm, they take up this new task in a last act of service to their hive. All these behaviors were discovered by Martin Lindauer in the 1950s when he devised an ingenious method to watch and track the scout bees in a swarm. He observed with an open mind and an attitude of wonder from the moment the bees left their hives at dawn to the moment they returned at sunset, letting the bees tell him their story without superimposing any preconceived ideas about insect intelligence.[4]

Approaching our relationship to other living things, as Lindauer did, with what Buddhists call the beginner's mind—observing without judgment or expectation—can help us avoid both the errors of assuming their experience of the world is just like ours or, on the other hand, assuming that only humans have emotion, self-awareness, and language. Both conclusions seem preposterous and highly unlikely when you stop to think about it. Taking the third path, staying open to mystery, to the possibility that our human minds will never completely comprehend how my cottonwood friend, or a bear, or a magpie experiences the world and relates to its kin, requires both imagination and being comfortable with uncertainty.

Making space in our lives to be in community with the natural world is difficult when we are bombarded with messages that encourage us to ignore our relationships with other creatures and urge us to center our own individual wants, needs, and desires. Many of us are trapped by a lifetime of conditioning and centuries of philosophical and religious thought that saturate every aspect of Western society, culture, and language. Thanks, Descartes. In modernity, our human-made world is almost entirely constructed to help us forget that we are just one small part of "nature." Our very senses have been commodified, corralled, and often dulled. The constant drumbeat everywhere reinforces a narrow, individualistic view of ourselves and diminishes the importance of our interdependence. But there are other ways and other cultural traditions that foster a more expansive worldview.

Language is a container for culture. It shapes our thoughts and perceptions. People who speak more than one language know that you learn to think differently and your perspective changes when seen through the lens of another way of describing the world. Linguists call this the Sapir-Whorf hypothesis, developed by Edward Sapir and Benjamin Whorf. They posited that "the structure of a language strongly influences or fully determines the way its native speakers perceive and reason about the world."[5] One example is the difference in perception between native speakers of noun-based languages like English and German, and those who speak verb-based languages prevalent among Indigenous and Asian peoples. The latter emphasize relationships and connections, while the former are more focused on categorizations and dualisms. Wade Davis described language as "the flash of the human spirit. It's a vehicle through which the soul of each particular culture comes into the world. Every language is an old growth forest of the mind, a watershed of thought, an ecosystem of spiritual and social possibilities."[6] Language can open doors to new ways of thinking, but it can also box us in.

Take the English word *wilderness*. The dictionary definition is "a tract or region uncultivated and uninhabited by human beings" or "an area essentially undisturbed by human activity together with its naturally developed life community" or "an empty or pathless region."[7] The word *nature* also excludes humans. Its definition is "the phenomena of the physical world collectively, including plants, animals, the landscape, and other features and products of the earth, as opposed to humans or human creations."[8]

Neither word exists in most Indigenous languages because the concept of a "natural world" or a "wilderness" entirely separate from the human world sounds like complete nonsense to most Native peoples. Indigenous cosmologies view human beings as a part of nature and see all living things in relationship with each other. In the essay "Listening to the Forest," Jeff Grignon and Robin Wall Kimmerer recount the story of an anthropologist who asked a Native person, "Do you go into the woods alone?" The Native person was flummoxed by this question, and the researcher was equally confused about why it was so difficult to answer. Each came to the question with his own cultural, ecological lens.[9] In fact, the Western concept of "nature" and "wilderness" is a lie. There is no place on Earth that hasn't been touched by human existence, and humans are a product of the natural world, completely embedded in and dependent on it. The idea of "pristine wilderness," in the way most European languages define it, has always been a myth.

If we go back far enough, our ancestors were all indigenous to someplace. Looking at the language of those times, we find words that describe more fully the connection between humans and their whole environment. In English there is the phrase *kith and kin* to mean our community of acquaintances, friends, and relatives. The two words originally had distinctive meanings. As naturalist and writer Lyanda Haupt points out in her book *Rooted*, *kin* is related to *kind*, as in "all the same kind," so might include all living beings, depending on your point of view. *Kith* originally meant the "known world" and related especially to one's native land and everything contained in it.[10] The word implied a deep relationship and intimacy with a place and all its inhabitants, including every plant and tree and bird and stone, and the human neighbors as well. As our disconnection from community and place grows and our culture changes, our language also forgets how to describe those atrophied relationships.

Cultures that retain their closeness to the land and their kinship with other living things have a different view of the place of humans in the world. Indigenous languages contain many words that embody the idea that "nature" is not separate from humans and that all beings are related and co-equal.

Enrique Salmon, a Rarámuri (Tarahumara) and head of the American Indian Studies program at Cal State University East Bay, explains this way of seeing the world in his essay "Kincentric Ecology," which centers on the meaning of *iwígara*.

> *The Rarámuri view themselves as an integral part of the life and place within which they live. There is among the Rarámuri a concept called iwígara, which encompasses many ideas and ways of thinking unique to the place with which the Rarámuri live. Rituals and ceremonies, the language, and, therefore, Rarámuri thought are influenced by the lands, animals, and winds with which they live. Iwígara is the total interconnectedness and integration of all life in the Sierra Madres, physical and spiritual. To say iwígara to a Rarámuri calls on that person to realize life in all its forms. The person recalls the beginning of Rarámuri life, origins, and relationships to animals, plants, the place of nurturing, and the entities to which the Rarámuri look for guidance.*

Dr. Salmon makes the case for adopting an Indigenous philosophy he calls kincentric ecology, or an "awareness that life in any environment is viable only when humans view the life surrounding them as kin." For the Rarámuri, all other beings were considered kin, or numatí, and the origins of their family ties are explained in their creation story. Dr. Salmon explains,

> *In a previous world, people were part plant. When the Rarámuri emerged into this world, many of those plants followed. They live today as humans of a different form. Peyote, datura, maize, morning*

glory, brazilwood, coyotes, crows, bears, and deer are all humans. Rarámuri feel related to these life-forms much as Euroamericans feel related to cousins and siblings. . . . A certain attachment results from knowing that some of your relatives are the life-forms that share your place with you. This belief influences one's sense of identity and thought/language.

Salmon goes on to argue that Indigenous cultural models of ecology, which prioritize relationships with the land and other living beings, can point the way to new and more sustainable conservation practices, ones that consider human cultures, "wilderness," and "nature" as part of the same family.[11]

Akiing is another word describing the relationship of land to people. It comes from Anishinaabeg and means "the land to which the people belong." When asked to elaborate on its meaning, Anishinaabe activist and writer Winona LaDuke explained, "It's also the land that we know . . . like, when I walk these woods, I know what's going to help me. I know where my medicines are. So, it's this relationship . . . it's a recognition of a mutual interdependence between you and the land."[12]

Hozhó is a Diné (Navajo) concept that refers to the interconnectedness between beauty, harmony and goodness in both the physical and spiritual realms that results in health and well-being for all beings. Diné poet and musician Lyla June Johnston describes it this way:

It is dawn. The sun is rising in the sky and my grandmother and I are singing prayers to the horizon. This morning, she's teaching me the meaning of hozhó. Although there's no direct translation from Diné Bizaad, the Navajo language, into English, every living being knows what hozhó means. For hozhó is every drop of rain. It is every leaf on every tree. It is your every eyelash. It is every feather on the blue bird's wing. Hozhó is undeniable beauty that surrounds us. Hozhó is remembering that you are part of the Earth's brilliance.[13]

Other examples include words like *orenda*, a Haudenosaunee word meaning a force that inhabits "all animate and inanimate natural objects as a transmissible spiritual energy." When looking for Native-authored articles on these concepts, I found very few. The most-cited article on orenda is from 1902, by a white anthropologist who calls the Haudenosaunee (Iroquois) "savage" repeatedly. He opens with the premise that man "at all times and in all lands learned he must struggle against the adverse conditions of his environment. Interpreted in terms of his self-centered philosophy, these unfavoring conditions were to the savage man the handiwork of mystic potence directed by the will of the environing bodies. . . . This conception persists up through barbarism and, albeit vestigially, into civilization."[14] The author could only see the world through his own lens of white human supremacy.

A google search for *orenda* comes back with a few more articles by white male anthropologists, and many companies that have stolen the word for its mystique, tarnishing its sacredness. The products bearing the name include supplements for menopausal women, swimming pool chemicals, a "glamping" experience in the Adirondack Mountains, a coffee maker, and a charter school. After trying and failing to kill Indigenous language outright, Western culture now resorts to appropriation to water down and destroy original meanings. Wade Davis contends that when languages die, we lose whole worldviews. Indigenous languages are not just dying, they're being murdered.

Writer and scientist Robin Wall Kimmerer, in the essay "Speaking of Nature," talks about the effects of forced residential schools, one of the main weapons used by European settlers to suffocate Indigenous culture and languages.

Within the walls of that school, the clipped syllables of English replaced the lush Potawatomi sounds of water splashing on rocks and wind in the trees, a language that emerged from the lands of the Great Lakes. Our language hovers at the edge of extinction, an endangered species of knowledge and wisdom dwindling away with the loss of every elder. Beyond the renaming of places, I think the most

profound act of linguistic imperialism was the replacement of a lan-
guage of animacy with one of objectification of nature, which renders
the beloved land as lifeless object, the forest as board feet of timber.[15]

It's truly difficult to understand the meaning of a word separately from its language and culture and place in time. I cannot say what exactly *iwígara* evokes for a Rarámuri person or what it felt like to a thirteenth-century Anglo-Saxon to hear the word *kith*. My understanding of these words is filtered through my own culture and experience. I cannot say how much they have in common, or how they are different, but it is clear that Western culture and languages have lost the meanings and the feelings that described the whole of Earth as an interconnected community in reciprocal relationship. The path forward is also a path back, to the time before we forgot our relationships with kith and kin.

The challenge to return to a different way of thinking of our place in the world can seem daunting. The first step is recognizing that modernity is based on the premise of anthropocentrism and the supremacy of Western culture. The colonial project was predicated on eliminating competing worldviews in favor of a justification for imperialism and empire building. Capitalism also relies on cultivating narcissistic individualism and myopic consumerism, ignoring the needs of kin in favor of feeding ever more esoteric personal desires.

Once we understand how language and culture can limit perception, we can start to retrain our minds to see the world in a new way. Start by cultivating an awareness of our integration with the world. We can recognize when and how we fall into human-centric and human-supremacist ways of thinking. We can develop new relationships with other living things and the land itself. We can create communities that encompass entire ecosystems, including people, plants, and animals. Finally, we can use our new sensibility to stop the destruction of languages, cultures, and non-Western ways of being, and instead learn what they have to teach us about fostering new relationships to create a healthier Earth for all its inhabitants.

Opening Our Eyes: From Human-Centric to Life-Centric

Changing thought patterns from individualistic to collective, and from human-centric to life-centric, is challenging when there is so little space in modern life for the more expansive frame. For most of us, the human-centric view is so ingrained, we barely think of it as such, but it's evident in almost every action we take: when we kill a scary spider in our bedroom, or use pesticides, or build roads, or decide what to plant in our garden, or plan our vacation, or scroll through carefully targeted social media ads, or think about what we want our city parks to look like. We nearly always consider first, and almost exclusively, the most convenient course of action for us humans. Thinking differently will take practice and pause, especially in societies that emphasize putting individual needs, wants, and desires above all else. On a scale developed by social psychologist Geert Hofstede, the United States, Australia, and the United Kingdom are the most individualistic countries, while Panama, Ecuador, and Guatemala are most collectivist.[16]

In his book about cultivating a more communal mindset, psychiatrist Dan Siegel describes how one's home culture can shape their sense of self and connection. He cites a study done with individuals from Japan and the United States who were given a picture of an aquarium and then asked to describe it. Those raised in the US were more likely to focus on attributes of individual fish, while the Japanese more commonly discussed the entire scene.[17] Many sociologists have blamed social media for society's increasing isolation, narcissistic focus, and the "death" of empathy, but the evidence is mixed. Studies from the US are more likely to correlate high social media use among young people with lower empathy scores, but in Europe, the research shows the opposite.[18] Perhaps the variation is attributable to a different background cultural emphasis on community and relationship.

Many writers and thinkers, including Dan Siegel, Thich Nhat Hanh, Enrique Salmon, and Robin Wall Kimmerer, have given us a wide range of guides for developing a greater sense of intraconnection, interbeing, and kinship, but all agree that rewilding our psyches depends on extricating ourselves from the boundaries that language and culture often impose. The roots are deep, from creation stories about severing ties with nature versus those that emphasize the symbiosis of all life systems, to the meaning of words we use every day, like *medicine, civilization, science,* or *primitive.* We catch ourselves talking about "developed nations" or referring possessively to "my property." Instead of acknowledging the other living things that share our space as relations, we objectify them with the pronoun *it.* Mother tongues impose lifelong conditioning; overcoming it takes a lot of intentional thinking and learning about other ways of seeing. The English language is objectifying and anthropocentric to its core. How can we invite the rest of the world to enter the conversation with us as equals?

A simple way to begin is a practice of mindfulness, just to notice how we are encouraged to unthinkingly objectify other beings. We can start by replacing the *it* in our minds with personal pronouns. Or as Kimmerer suggests, we could create an entirely new language. She asks "Can we unlearn the language of objectification and throw off colonized thought? Can we make a new world with new words?" She considers the word *Aakibmaadiziiwin,* which means "a being of the earth" in Potawatomi, the language of her ancestors.

> *With full recognition and celebration of its Potawatomi roots, might we hear a new pronoun at the beginning of the word, from the "aaki" part that means land? Ki to signify a being of the living earth. Not he or she, but ki. So that when the robin warbles on a summer morning, we can say, "Ki is singing up the sun." Ki runs through the branches on squirrel feet, ki howls at the moon, ki's branches sway in the pine-scented breeze, all alive in our language as in our world.*[19]

We can begin to practice every day an awareness of how our language shapes our thinking, and cultivate a curiosity about other languages and words, and even start to create new language. We can also support work to preserve native languages, like that being done at the Indigenous Language Institute in Santa Fe. Although the task of decolonizing our language and learning to "unobjectify" the world around us is a critical first step, it won't mean much unless our new way of seeing is translated into action. Connection to place is at the root of rebuilding our relationships with the land and our neighbors, humans and others, with whom we share it.

Rekindling Reciprocal Relationships

Researchers recently mapped the habitats of different bear family groups in British Columbia. They were surprised to see territories of distinct genetically related bears directly overlap the map of Indigenous language groups. The discovery came as no surprise to Native people. Different ecosystems, or nations, embodied the humans and the bears and the trees and all the beings in the same family. They were all equal citizens of the community. The discovery was astonishing to non-Indigenous people because these concepts are so strange to us. In recent history, Euro-Americans have two principal ways of relating to the land. It is either seen as something to serve humans by ownership, cultivation, extraction or subjugation, or seen as something precious to be preserved as "wilderness," separated from humans. The ancient way of seeing the land and everything in it as family—genetically and biologically connected —is foreign to most of us indoctrinated in modern Western culture.

In mainstream society, decisions about land use are made based on what is pleasing, convenient, or "good" for humans. Everything from lawns to dams comes from this view. Our world is less often seen through the lens of relationship than it is through that of domination and exploitation. Vine Deloria Jr., one of the best-known Native American authors and activists of the twentieth century, pointed out that Indigenous cosmologies emphasize responsibilities and obligations— to the land, to the creatures that inhabit it, and to each other. In contrast, modern European cultures, having themselves been largely divested of their Indigenous roots, have come to emphasize individual rights. The former worldview is more conducive to creating bonds, like those mycelial connections binding together all the trees in a forest. The latter creates separation and competition.

Most Indigenous cultures learn this symbiotic way of thinking from childhood, from creation stories that emphasize interdependence with the earth. Western cultures also have ancient stories and mythology about our relations with the natural world. The story of St. Francis and the wolf is one example. In 1220, in the small Italian town of Gubbio, a fierce wolf started attacking livestock and then the people of the town. Many people tried to kill the wolf, but he was too powerful and struck them all down and ate them. St. Francis of Assisi approached the wolf's den and offered him a deal. If the wolf would agree to stop devouring the villagers, the town would ensure the wolf was fed and could live in peace the rest of his days. The wolf accepted and lived in harmony with the villagers until his death. St. Francis negotiated a coexistence that considered both the needs of the wolf and the villagers. When the wolf died a few years later, the villagers honored him with a sacred burial under the Church of St. Francis of the Peace (in the 1800s, the skeleton of a wolf was actually discovered under the church). Although Christian religions may see a parable about the power of God to subdue nature, we can read it differently. In the light of St. Francis's later teachings about the sanctity of all creatures and the presence of God in all of creation, the message can be a concept similar to orenda. Francis saw himself as just one part of nature and considered other living things as his kin.

How might we use our own history and mythology, along with the teachings from other cultures, to rekindle that old Anglo-Saxon idea of kith? I am privileged to live in northern New Mexico, in a community that retains the idea of a commons, or shared resources that we are all obligated to caretake. Caring for our acequia system keeps our valley ecosystem vibrant and diverse, binds our community together, and also binds us to the land, even though few of us depend on the ditch for our main sustenance anymore. In gathering together, we share stories and build relationships. We learn to care for each other and the land, and develop intimacies that can only come from working side by side.

In a conversation with Enrique Salmon, we talked about time he spent working with acequia communities in northern New Mexico and southern Colorado. He recalled "how those descendants from the colonists that came with Don Juan Onate in 1598, they, over time, became indigenous to that whole area in Northern NM and Southern Colorado. Rio Arriba, as they referred to it. So, it's not impossible for an entire community like that to become indigenous, and it's about recognizing again the inner workings of a particular ecosystem or landscape." I am reminded again of the word *querencia* in Spanish, which is like *kith*. It describes a sanctuary where one feels safe, from which one can draw strength, where one is most at home and deeply connected.

Perhaps we cannot "become indigenous" in the same way we would be if we still inhabited the same land our ancestors lived in and cultivated for centuries. It might be possible though to become naturalized citizens of an adopted homeland, along with other invasive but sometimes helpful species. Robin Wall Kimmerer offers those of us who are immigrants a beautiful model to follow with a metaphor using two nonnative plant species, kudzu and plantain. Plants like kudzu come to dominate, choking out all the indigenous species, growing unchecked, and using up resources with no regard for others. In contrast, plantain, which the Anishinaabe call "white man's footsteps," fit into the landscape and became useful to the people, offering itself as food and medicine. Kimmerer concludes, "Being naturalized to place means to live as if this is the land that feeds you, as if these are the streams from which you drink, that build your body and fill your spirit. To become naturalized is to know that your ancestors lie in this ground. Here you will give your gifts and meet your responsibilities. To become naturalized is to live as if your children's future matters, to take care of the land as if our lives and the lives of all our relatives depend on it. Because they do."[20]

How can we be like the plantain and build community with other humans and the natural world around us? We might start from a place of curiosity, by learning to identify the beings with whom we share our space. We could do this not in a competitive way, like some bird-watchers do, collecting notches in their belt and keeping lists of how many things they have seen or "captured" in images, but with the Buddhist's beginner's mind, open to wonder. Naming and categorizing can be an act of domination, or an act of relationship and connection—the difference lies in an empathetic mindset and a desire to see the world from other perspectives. We can go further than just learning names by observing habits and learning histories and names in local dialects or Indigenous languages. We can use all our senses, learning to recognize the smell left behind when a bear has ambled through in the night looking for windfall apples, or the distinctive calls of the birds in our neighborhood. We can do this also with the land itself and geographical features, like mountains and lakes, in our surroundings.

I have a kind of game I play with the birds that I share my space with. I observe the flight patterns of each one and imagine how I would see them if the sky were an ocean. The magpies fly with an elegant breaststroke, the crows and ravens glide over the currents like sleek sailboats. The doves dog-paddle and the bushtits bob and bounce like dolphins playing in surf. The turkey vulture looks like an old, barely seaworthy skiff, tottering in the distance. Learning their patterns makes it easier for me to recognize them in the same way I can recognize an old friend at a distance just by their silhouette and their walk.

Dr. Salmon gives an assignment to students in his America Indian Science class to observe the sun or the moon every week at the same time of day. They are asked to record both objective data, like temperature, degree from the horizon, weather conditions, but also to journal about their experiences and feelings in the moment of observation. For many of his urban students, it becomes a practice of mindful connection, orienting them to the natural world in ways they had never before experienced. They notice variations in the colors of the sunset seen for the first time, or a certain elderly couple who walk the same path holding hands each evening.[21]

We can all follow this practice in our own ways. In my backyard, I created a small pond ecosystem ringed by rocks with a few steps leading down to murky waters that churn with life most of the year. If I am sufficiently quiet and calm, the other creatures forget I am there. They no longer see me as a threat, but part of their community. I watch as the garter snake sits motionless on lily pads, alert to the possibility of dragonfly nymph or young salamander feast. Dragonflies buzz around looking for food and mates, sometimes landing on my head as a good high perch. Birds will alight just a few feet away to bathe and drink in the fountain that gurgles up from one of the stones. I start to notice new sensations, like the feeling of pond muck between my toes, or an insect or birdcall I hadn't heard before. Find your own place to sit and observe and be still. See what happens, what you feel, what you sense, what you notice that you've never seen or felt or heard before.

Sometimes we can turn these quiet moments into opportunities to create relationships, and like the plantain, find ways to offer our gifts to the other beings in our community. We can start to notice what our relations need and sometimes provide for them, maybe by curing a coyote of mange or helping a cottonwood tree live a few more years. We might find that by entering into this community of other beings, we ourselves are also nourished and healed.

Those who live in urban environments might protest that these practices are harder there, but the natural world is always all around us. We are limited in ways to connect to nature only by our own imaginations. My friend Dan was raised on the Tulalip Nation in Washington State and his mother was an elder and archivist for the tribe. When we talk about different cultures' concepts of connection to place, he nods in recognition and shares that his querencia is the community where he grew up. For decades now, he has made his home in urban Seattle and has been witness to the unchecked gentrification and development that is destroying much of the city's residential tree canopy, among other ills. A few years ago he turned a former parking spot in his front yard into a "nanoforest," in part as an art project and also a political statement. It's a beautiful little niche of native plants and serves as a home and forage for urban wildlife, as well as a reminder to his neighbors of what is being lost. Another friend in Cleveland lives close to an abandoned corner of a city park. He asked permission to "adopt" the space and has removed invasive weeds and trash and started cultivating native plants. In just over a year, he's noticed many local species have sprouted up that he didn't intentionally introduce; they just found the welcoming space he created and considered it an invitation to join the community.

These are just two examples of practices that build relationship and create ways to be useful to our kin. Small ideas like these can start to create healthier ecosystems, but to create lasting social and environmental change, we must go further. We must ask, How can we leverage these relationships to go beyond individual actions and develop ethical frameworks that will help us build a more sustainable society on a larger scale?

What Kind of Ancestor?

In our quest to recall ancient ways of thinking about our place in the world, and to center rekindled relationships with our kin, we will need to create new ways of evaluating almost everything we do. We require a set of ethics that considers all life as equally valuable. Again, we can look to both Western and Indigenous cultures for examples.

In his essay "The *Akiing* Ethic," nature writer John Hausdoerffer explores the connections between noted conservationist Aldo Leopold's "land ethic" and the Anishinaabe concept of "akiing." In the last chapter of *A Sand County Almanac*, Leopold argues for "changing the role of *Homo sapiens* from conqueror of the land-community to plain member and citizen of it." In Hausdoerffer's words, "Leopold challenges readers to measure right and wrong, in all aspects of life, based on whether or not their reactions as landowner, consumers or citizens 'preserve' the 'integrity, stability, and beauty' of the 'community.'" Hausdoerffer visits White Earth Nation, home of the Anishinaabe people, to seek the counsel of activist and author Winona LaDuke, who advises against "drawing too many analogies between Anishinaabeg lifeway and Western notions." In the end, he concludes that akiing is a more evolved and reciprocal relationship with the land, inviting "humans to become cocreators in addition to preservers of the 'wild process.'" He writes, "I found far more than a connection between Leopold's hope for a land ethic and LaDuke's call for native justice. I learned a view of land—*akiing*—that challenges, strengthens, and surpasses Leopold's ideas."[22]

While at White Earth, Hausdoerffer is asked to consider, "What kind of ancestor do you want to be?" The query echoes the seven generations principle, from Haudenosaunee philosophy, which requires every decision about resources and relationships to take into consideration the effects for seven generations. The period is the "wingspan" of a human life, considering that my existence will touch my great-grandparents' lives and also the lives of my great-grandchildren.

To meet the modern challenges of climate change and environmental degradation, the lifeways of many cultures will have to be woven into a new ethical framework for our times. We might evolve these ideas into a new kind of precautionary principle, one that gives us time and space to pause and consider the ramifications of our actions on all living things and on Gaia herself.

The precautionary principle states that it's not enough for a proposal or a policy or new technology to simply "lack evidence of harm"—it must be actively proven as "not harmful." The burden of proof is shifted. The new process or chemical is "guilty until proven innocent," especially when there is a dearth of scientific evidence about possible harms. The principle recommends extreme caution, review, and proceeding slowly when introducing new, potentially harmful innovations to ensure they are "not harmful to humans." What if we extended the precaution to mean "not harmful to communities of living things and the land," and extended our timeframe for seven generations?

These ideas may seem radical, but our times call for radical solutions. We will not survive if we continue to behave as though human beings exist within a separate bubble, divorced from the natural world. We are nature, nature is us, and when we harm it, we harm ourselves. The only path with a future is a path that leads us back, to the time before we created separations and divisions with our kin and the land we inhabit. Only this journey, toward a reintegration and reunion with the natural world, will give us *Homo sapiens* purpose and authenticity from which we can begin to act collectively for renewal and healing. We can begin by using some of the examples and inspiration described here. We will not be alone, as there are organizations and movements in every part of the United States and the globe that are already applying these ethics and practices to create a better world.

Possible Futures

The unleashed power of the atom has changed everything
except our thinking. Thus, we are drifting toward catastrophe
beyond conception. We shall require a substantially new
manner of thinking if mankind is to survive.

—ALBERT EINSTEIN

The past couple of days, I've seen the same coyote prancing through the orchard behind my house in the dawn light. I came upon him yesterday as I stepped out the front door to walk the dogs, only thirty feet away. He stopped and stared at us, unmoving and unfazed, for a good minute. We paused and regarded him. I wondered what was going through his mind as he considered the three of us—my two pups on leashes, one straining to be let free for a romp with this new friend. Does he know how lucky he has it to live in a place where his coyote clan can, for the most part, harmoniously coexist with humans? Where the occasional loss of a chicken or even a pet cat is chalked up to the price we pay to be on friendly terms? Does he appreciate the offerings I leave in the compost pile—broth-soaked vegetables and, most recently, a chicken carcass? Later in the day, a neighbor will come over and help me get my trash to the dump. I'll tell him about the coyote and he'll remark that he's seen the same one, he thinks, prowling around the chicken coop. He'll bring a gift of elk jerky and I'll offer up some freshly made stock in thanks. It's late winter as I write this and the weather is turning warmer. This is breeding season for the coyotes, the time of year when they are most vocal, and when their songs seem most varied. The snowpack this past winter has been scant, not nearly enough to fill the acequia in spring, and just a few gray patches persist in the northern shade of the house. Still we will gather in a few weeks for the annual ditch cleaning as we do every year, hope and communal spirit triumphing over pessimism and isolation.

I give thanks for my community of beings, which seems more anomalous and rare with every passing day. The news tells us the planet is growing ever hotter with no signs the trend will be mitigated. Refugees of climate catastrophes and war, both caused by us humans, amass at the borders of nearly every wealthy country. I wonder if our communal habits can be sustained through the perilous times ahead of us. The worst drought in twelve centuries plagues much of the West, and the Rio Grande seems to run thinner and dry earlier every year. Will our community continue our rituals when they seem more performative than practical? All around our enclave, the sixth mass extinction continues apace, wiping out species faster than we can know or even name them. Natural disasters are destroying whole towns. Entire ecosystems are dying or being irrevocably changed. The COVID pandemic has claimed over five million lives worldwide and spawned another epidemic of grief that will reverberate for generations, this on top of the widespread grief over the loss of the earth as we have known it. And most recently, conflicts in Sudan, the Congo, Ukraine, and Gaza continue with almost no regard for the sanctity of life, while fears abound of another world war igniting from the disputes.

We Are Doing It Wrong

The outlook is bleak in our Anthropocene moment. We *sapiens* can't seem to find a way to get along with our fellow beings or even among ourselves. Human alteration of the environment is everywhere. No corner of the earth is untouched or unchanged—every place seems threatened. Humans, animals, and even plants are migrating to find more hospitable environs, but their efforts are mostly thwarted—every spot is already occupied. We are all seeking safe haven to weather this storm and swiftly realizing that the elements all living beings require— like clear water, breathable air, healthy food, shelter and space—are growing scarcer and ever more precious.

Scientists tell us the changes are accelerating faster even than their already dire models predicted. We hear reports that to stave off disaster we need to act by 2030, just a few years away. We are told we must cut our carbon emissions in half by then, and by half again every decade until the end of the century. In desperation and guilt, we grasp at the straws of individual behavior change. We might recycle more, drive a little less, set the thermostat a smidge lower, go to a protest or two—nothing too inconvenient. It all seems so futile, but what else is there to be done?

Most of us agree we're doing it wrong, we're on the wrong path. The human and the natural worlds seem to be breaking apart, disintegrating, before our very eyes. Our leaders and systems are failing us. Polarization, division, and degradation are the themes of our times. We know we're stuck, but the consensus stops there. We can't seem to agree about how to get unstuck and get on the right path, if there even is one right path. We stay mired in conflicts and argument, failing to find the swift and productive way forward we all desperately desire. It's as if we're all trapped on a speeding train headed for the edge of the cliff and none of us know how to stop it.

The big conclusions are inescapable. In order to stave off impending disaster, we must reduce, and eventually eliminate, our use of fossil fuels. Opinions about how to accomplish this vary widely, from those who hope for a single technological fix that allows us to continue living almost exactly how we always have, to those who say we must completely retool everything about how our society works and how we live on the earth. Either extreme seems inaccessible to us average humans trying to survive day to day, so we read the news of the most recent wildfire or dying coral reef or lost species or refugee crisis and become increasingly depressed. The term *eco-grief* has been coined to refer to the sense of loss from learning about the scale of ongoing environmental destruction, or the mourning for ecosystems and landscapes and nature that have been destroyed, or a feeling of hopelessness that sets in when we feel helpless to effect real change.[1]

Going back to the analogy of people drowning in the river, most of us know the river is dangerous, but for many of us, it is also unavoidable. At times we all feel swept away in that river and desperate to find a way out. Whether or not we think we're currently drowning, we are constantly aware of the river just a few steps away. We may not be homeless or living on top of a Superfund site, but even the wealthiest among us are susceptible to the toxic effects of the environment we've created. The air we all breathe in our cities is so polluted it kills an estimated 100,000 Americans every year.[2] A 2011 study estimated that 245,000 people die yearly in the United States as a result of social factors like inequality, racism and poverty.[3] Worldwide, the WHO estimates one in four deaths are linked to environmental factors.[4]

A Sense of Futility

In moments of desperation, we are vulnerable to snake oil salesmen offering simple panaceas. We get seduced by the vast wellness industry into believing that if we just do a few simple things, like eating only organic foods, or exercising every day, or taking a few supplements, or moving to the countryside, we'll be insulated from all that toxicity we see affecting others. These tonics are often distractions from what is most important and necessary for the well-being of ourselves and Earth. What if instead of working individually to become the best, most beautiful version of ourselves, we worked together to build healthy communities and ecosystems and to heal at least some of the damage that's been inflicted? Where would we even start that kind of project?

The TV show *The Good Place* was premised on the idea that it's impossible to "be good" in modern society because unintended consequences will always undermine even the most noble efforts. In the show, it's revealed that to get to heaven, or the Good Place, humans need to accrue a certain number of do-gooder points, but for over 500 years not a single person has managed to reach the required total. One man living off the grid in Canada has figured out the system and tried to calculate all his actions and behaviors so that he will be rewarded in the afterlife, but even he is destined for the Bad Place/Hell instead. Almost every "good" thing he tries to do results in some harm. An example is proffered of a man living in the year 1500 who gave roses to his mother on her birthday and earned 1000 points. When a man does the same thing in 2010, he loses 1000 points because the roses were grown with slave labor on deforested and colonized land, doused with pesticides, flown thousands of miles, and trucked to the florist.

We all feel trapped by constrained choices. We must drive cars to get to work or use fossil fuels to heat our houses. We crave the newest technology and may need it for our jobs, but at the same time, we become distressed reading about conflict mineral mining in Africa and South America. We accept the plastic bag for our purchases at the convenience store or drive through the fast-food joint on road trips because other options are unworkable. We keep marching down the path that we know is wrong while trying to mitigate as much as we can, but somehow we're all stuck in the same lockstep, just going at slightly different speeds. We feel trapped and powerless to free ourselves.

Imagining the Future

In *The Future We Choose: Surviving the Climate Crisis*, the architects of the 2015 Paris Agreement, Christiana Figueres and Tom Rivett-Carnac, describe the two possible futures. One is inevitable if we continue our current ways; the other is an unwritten book, open to our creativity and experimentation. Figueres and Rivett-Carnac call them "the world we are creating" and "the world we must create." They warn that if we continue apace without shifting direction, "human misery would be high, biodiversity would be decimated, and . . . our children would live in a world that is constantly deteriorating with no possible recuperation."[5] David Wallace-Wells tries to shake us out of our state of denial by sharing a dark story of where our current path leads according to the best data and modeling we have. He starts his book *The Uninhabitable Earth* with the words "it's worse, much worse than you think." In the subsequent two hundred pages he enumerates the many dire consequences foretold by scientists if we allow the Earth to warm by more than two degrees Celsius, ranging from the decreased nutritional content of food crops to killer heat waves and droughts, to plagues, and finally to geopolitical power struggles over resources causing a constant state of war. All these devastating consequences of our current path should sound familiar to anyone who has perused a newspaper recently.

Facts can be debated, and the theories that require understanding of probability curves or economic theory or thermohaline circulation can be hard to apply to quotidian life. Fiction writers are increasingly filling that gap between what the scientific models predict and what our imaginations can hold. "Science fiction is a way to practice the future together," writes adrienne maree brown,[6] and so many storytellers have taken on the challenge of showing us those possible futures. Kim Stanley Robinson opens *The Ministry for the Future* with an apocalyptic scene: an aid worker in India watches helplessly as an entire town perishes around him, the result of an overpowering heatwave.[7] Octavia Butler predicted another kind of apocalypse in *Parable of the Sower*. In a futuristic story becoming more and more plausible, she foresaw a world where the rule of law has broken down, resources are scarce, and drug addiction and violence run rampant.[8] She focuses her tale on a small band of resilient humans who set out to find a safe refuge amid the devastation. In *Migrations*, Charlotte McConaghy imagines a world where nearly all the wildlife is gone, a subtler kind of apocalypse. Her protagonist risks life and limb to follow the last few arctic terns on their final annual journey spanning the whole of the globe from the Arctic Circle to the Antarctic.[9]

Judging from the news, we are inching (or maybe hurtling) toward the future foretold by Robinson, Butler, McConaghy, and the scientists in Wallace-Wells's cautionary tome. Growing inequality is deepening distrust, division, social isolation, and societal disintegration. Our society increasingly looks like the landscape described in *Parable of the Sower*, where the ultrarich can wall themselves off in gated communities, paying for their own private security, power systems, and even firefighters, as we are seeing now every summer when the California wildfire season inevitably arrives. The rest of us are left to depend on crumbling public infrastructure and feel increasingly vulnerable.

While many have predicted what will happen if we don't correct course, in his work of speculative nonfiction *The Future Earth*, Eric Holthaus instead describes what we could achieve if we listen to the scientists and the activists and act collectively in the interest of our own well-being and Earth's. "Success on climate change," he observes, "where it can exist, will look like democracy. To build a sustainable just world for the next century, everyone will have to participate—especially those who have been excluded from the political process for far too long. An inclusive society is a just society, in which we all listen to one other with genuine care."[10]

Ursula K. Le Guin offers us a parable for the consequences of our choices in *Always Coming Home*, in which the two paths are embodied in the stories of two different cultures living in California eons after modern civilization has collapsed. A future anthropologist named Pandora is the narrator and fictional author of the book, which reads like an anthropological study. She describes the Kesh people, who live lightly on the land in small, self-governing, pacifist, egalitarian communities. In contrast, Pandora's own people in the "mainstream" society are patriarchal, authoritarian, militaristic, and imperialistic. Pandora clearly prefers the healthier and more joyful lifestyle of the Kesh and offers the book to her contemporaries as a protest and counterpoint. Le Guin's cautionary tale is not hard to decipher. Indeed, critics of *Always Coming*

Home point out that many of the details of Kesh life are taken from anthropological descriptions of Indigenous American communities.[11]

In all these depictions of the future, the only commonality is change. A different future is coming, that is certain. We cannot turn back the clock or undo all the damage that has been done. According to the bleakest predictions, it may even be too late to prevent warming past the dangerous two-degree Celsius mark that would make much of Earth uninhabitable. We must adapt to an unknown future while we concurrently work to mitigate the greatest predicted harms. How might we shift course and avoid the tunnel in front of us that leads to more disconnection, exclusion, conflict, and the breakdown of democratic systems of governance? Listening to the storytellers might give us the clues we require to change course and choose the way that leads toward inclusiveness, collaboration, participation, and cohesive community.

If all the dire predictions seem overwhelming, it's because they absolutely are. The bright futures hoped for by Holthaus and Figueres and Rivett-Carnac feel entirely out of reach in our current political climate. A sense of futility leads us to focus on our immediate surroundings, on the things we can affect—ourselves and our families and communities. In the previous chapter I talked about the changes in attitude we can make in the way we see and relate to the world. Creating relationships with other living things brings them into our families and communities as kin. Practicing being in relationship, working to get to know *all* our neighbors (human or not) will build empathy, trust, and an ethic of common good. These shifts are necessary, but not sufficient. To bring about significant change, we must act from this new sense of kinship.

Centering Well-Being for All Creatures

In the first chapters, I made the case that human beings have gone from thousands of different ways of doing things and living in the world to being stuck in one destructive pattern that's killing us and the earth. What if there isn't one path that leads away from our species demise? What if there are thousands of paths? How might we experiment with different ways of healthier living? Rather than hoping for some miracle to save us, could we combine all our ways of knowing, from both Indigenous science and Western technologies, to find the paths that are the most sustainable and healing for all of us?

We already have a lot of data about how to do this. Let's try a thought experiment: If you and I were alien beings and I gave you a gift of humans to nurture and a giant terrarium, what would the care instructions look like? What kind of world would you want to build for them, for all of us, if we could start anew, applying all that we've learned in the past few millennia about what humans and other living things need to thrive?

We humans do best when we have meaningful connections with other humans, when we have time and space for contemplation and grief and creativity and joy and exercise, in community and alone. We thrive in more egalitarian societies, devoid of prejudices and stark economic inequalities. We need clean water and air, and healthy soils that can grow nutritious foods. We also do much better when we feel integrated with the natural world all around us. We are interdependent on a rich and diverse biome of living organisms, inside and outside our bodies. The Lakota distinguish humans from other beings not because they are superior but because they are the most interdependent, requiring help from all other species to keep warm, to eat, for shelter, and for every necessary function of life.

Zooming out and considering what the planet needs to thrive, to support us and other living things, it's a lot of the same things. Gaia also needs rich biodiversity, healthy soils, and clean water and air to thrive. Every interconnected ecosystem between our own bodies and the whole Earth is dependent on reciprocal and symbiotic relationships between all the beings inhabiting them.

Building Arks

The idea of "arks" as a metaphorical response to our turbulent future was coined by fellow New Mexican writer and lifelong conservationist

William deBuys. DeBuys believes it's too late to preserve much of the old earth, as species go extinct at startling rates every year and whole ecosystems are snuffed out on a daily basis. But maybe we can still preserve some parts, and those can be centers of resilience and rebirth after the storm subsides. The second dictionary definition of *ark*, after Noah's boat, is "something that affords protection and safety." The third is "the sacred chest representing to the Hebrews the presence of God among them."[12] Combining all three, an ark might be thought of as a sacred vessel that provides refuge and safe passage.

Contemplating the significance of the word *ark* for our times leads me to another word mentioned before in these pages, one that has special significance in northern New Mexico. It comes from the Spanish of the fifteenth and sixteenth centuries, when New Mexico was being colonized by conquistadores and outcasts from Spain. The word *querencia* originated as a bullfighting term for the place in the ring where the bull feels safest, where he can gather his strength, where he feels indefatigable. The place is different for each bull, and part of the job of a skilled matador is to identify his foe's querencia and keep him from accessing this place of resilience. Ironically, this is exactly what the original settlers tried to do to the Indigenous people they found living in this land when they arrived—they destroyed their querencia and displaced the original peoples to make their own communities and safe havens. These patterns continue today—the needs of a society dependent on fossil fuels and consumerism take precedence over the sacred spaces that provide sustenance and strength to humans and other beings.

The word *querencia* has evolved to mean more than a physical place and can refer to anything that provides resilience or power. Another meaning is a space where one can be their most authentic self. A querencia can be a kind of landscape, a work of art, or a community. Thinking about these two concepts together, arks and querencias, led me to start imagining what these spaces would look like for whole ecosystems, whole communities of living things. What if we intentionally worked to create querencias for both coyotes and humans, where all of us feel safe and secure and able to be our true selves? Could these safe havens serve as refuges as we traverse the tumultuous times ahead? If we look around, more compassionate and connected ways of living are continually being invented all over the world.

In the previous chapters, I've described some places that fit the definition of querencia. The Greek island of Ikaria is clearly a querencia to those who have a connection to the place. The Near West Side of Cleveland is another, and I continue to draw strength from the spirit of that community and the ties I formed there even though I moved away almost twenty years ago. My village in New Mexico could fit the definition. The community includes not only the humans but all living things and provides an ancient system of sharing resources that might help us better weather the coming storm—coyotes and humans alike. Our mayordomo manages our water resources to share with the homeowners, but also with the river itself. He carefully controls the distribution to ensure that the seasonal flow persists as long as possible and is equitably divided between people and wildlife. I feel at home and interdependent here, with my animal and human neighbors, even when we don't see eye to eye. This kind of living isn't without conflict, but when a basis of trust and understanding exists, the disputes are more easily resolved.

Looking around your own city or neighborhood, you can likely find examples where people are coming together in innovative ways to build connections between humans and nature, healing relationships and landscapes, and creating new ways of living on the earth by reviving and remembering old knowledge. Part of building arks also must be acknowledging and understanding the trauma that a place and a people have suffered in the past. The healing of wounds isn't easy, but it's a prerequisite to creating well-being and resilience.

Healing Wounds

The town of Española is situated between its more famous neighbors of Santa Fe and Taos. It was the original epicenter of the colonial occupation of the lands now known as New Mexico and is still surrounded by several Tewa-speaking Pueblo nations, including Ohkay Owingeh, Nambe, Tesuque, Pojoaque, Santa Clara (Kha'p'oe Owingeh), and San Idelfonso (Po-Woh-Geh Owingeh). The whole of the Rio Grande Valley was subject to brutal massacres and subjugation in waves of conquest, first by the Coronado expedition and later by Juan de Oñate. Some of the first and most brutal massacres in the lands that became the United States occurred here. In 1540 Coronado stormed up the Rio Grande Valley from Mexico and took control of one of the Pueblos for his vast expedition that included at least two thousand people and thousands of horses, cows, mules, and pigs. They stayed for two years, commandeering housing and food for themselves and their livestock and wiping out entire communities of anyone who protested. Later, in 1598, Oñate arrived and again demanded subjugation of the Indigenous people, including slave labor to build settlements and churches for the invaders. When the men of Acoma resisted, Oñate indiscriminately killed and enslaved hundreds of them and famously sentenced men over twenty-five to have one of their feet cut off as an example to the rest.

In the century that followed Oñate's brutal occupation, the Spanish sought not only to enslave and dominate the Indigenous people but to eliminate their entire culture. Missionaries demanded allegiance to their Christian God and forbade ceremonies, dances, and other displays of traditional spirituality. This intentional genocide of both a people and their cultural knowledge continued until, in 1675, the arrest of forty-seven Pueblo healers, or "medicine men," was ordered by the Spanish governor. Four Indigenous men were sentenced to death by hanging, while the others were imprisoned and publicly tortured. Upon hearing the news of these atrocities, a large contingent of Pueblo leaders converged on Santa Fe and demanded the release of the men. One of these, from Ohkay Owingeh, was Popé.

Once he was released, Popé retreated far from Santa Fe to Taos, and spent five years organizing the forty-six Pueblo towns along the

Rio Grande to rise up in the Pueblo Revolt of 1680. Their rebellion successfully drove the Spanish settlers out of the area for twelve years, until the reconquest by Diego de Vargas in 1692. To this day, many places in New Mexico carry the names of Coronado, Oñate, and De Vargas, but almost none are named for Popé or the other leaders of the Pueblo Revolt. To understand what the commemoration of these events means to the Indigenous people here, imagine for a moment that Hitler had won and the descendants of Jewish people had to live on streets and patronize businesses named for him and Goebbels and Hess.

This history is carried in the DNA of both the Indigenous people, who still inhabit their ancestral lands here, and in the descendants of the Spanish settlers, as well as within the land itself. To heal old wounds, these stories must be retold, acknowledged and confronted, and this work is exactly what Tewa Women United is doing in the Española Valley today.

From their website, Tewa Women United is a "multicultural and multiracial organization founded and led by Native women." The name *Tewa Women United* comes from the Tewa words *wi don gi mu*, which can be translated as "we are one" in mind, heart, and in the spirit of love for all. One of the most inspiring among many projects the group has led is the Española Healing Foods Oasis. TWU took an abandoned and barren site between city administrative buildings and a small park and transformed it in a few years to a publicly accessible garden and "food forest" with Native medicinal herbs and plants, a beautiful winding path, and a natural rainwater collection system. What was once a dusty slope where runoff from the parking lots above swept away all the topsoil—and any seedling that hoped to find purchase there—is now a lush, inviting garden for community gatherings. Using Indigenous permaculture practices and employing a multicultural workforce of volunteers, the Healing Foods Oasis now boasts more than 200 native plant and tree species. Weekend community planting and harvesting days attract locals who build relationships with each other and learn new ways to connect to the land. The communal space is home for pollinators and birds who have returned to make a rich, biodiverse ecosystem shared by humans and all other living creatures. All the beings, humans or birds or bees, are invited to take what they need from the garden for their sustenance.

Start Where You Are

In your own community, or nearby, you can likely find groups engaged in similar projects. Look for work centered on healing old traumas and the scars that remain in the land as well as in the DNA of the descendants of prior and current inhabitants. The work begins by building relationships rooted in the idea that all life is sacred and worth preserving, and then finding ways of living together that honor all creatures.

Many books, like Holthaus's *Future Earth* and Figueres and Rivett-Carnac's *The Future We Choose*, close with a list of suggestions for further action. Inevitably, these are aimed at individuals. Holthaus suggests becoming more aware and mindful of our ecosystems and the natural world, and then engaging others by talking about climate change, going to a protest, or running for office. Figueres and Rivett-Carnac have a ten-point action plan including "letting go" of past patterns of consumerism and dependence on fossil fuels, facing your grief while imagining a new future, learning and talking to others about the truth of climate change, planting trees, engaging politically, and becoming a better and more engaged consumer. Although these suggestions may be a start, they can feel insufficient. Many of us feel that we've been practicing these activities for years, and all around us things seem to be getting worse, not better.

Rather than more lists of individual actions, how can we shift focus to the collective work of fostering communities of care centered on healing and protecting? This work is hard and requires openness and humility. Part of becoming more grounded and connected to the earth is also learning the history of places that hold meaning for you and understanding the meaning they may hold for others. More often than not, those who have been oppressed, whose ancestors held critical knowledge about different ways of living on the earth, will have to lead these efforts, and the rest of us will need to follow and learn.

Some guidelines are helpful when embarking on such work. First, don't assume that you have to do it all yourself. If you look around your community, you will likely find many efforts already happening. Look especially for projects led by Black, Indigenous, and other people of color. Join with these actions humbly and be open to new answers and different ways of seeing the world. Listen. Be vulnerable. Ask yourself if some beings are being excluded or forgotten, and if so, invite them to the table. Learn solidarity and collaboration, and let go of defensiveness and ego.

It's clear we can't avoid the storm, but if we are open and curious, we'll find there are many spaces and projects and ideas that offer refuge and hope for the future. Collectively building centers of compassion and resilience has the potential to protect humans and other living things as we confront our turbulent times. We can all find ways to participate in these forms of modern-day ark building.

Most days, the task of transforming our society seems too daunting. Feelings of defeat are inevitable. Exactly for that reason, having the support of a community becomes so critical. When considering where to focus our attention, we feel forced to choose between individual actions that feel too small, or huge technological or policy fixes that seem so far beyond our own sphere of influence. Maybe there is a third option. We can join together to build places of resilience, arks that provide refuge and safe passage, querencias from which all living things can draw strength and feel safe.

Willam deBuys describes it this way:

We know things will get worse before they get better. The momentum of climate change guarantees it, to say nothing of the assured increase of human population by several billions more. Such prospects behoove us to become latter-day Noahs. We need to build arks, vehicles to carry the beauty and diversity of the Earth's present creation across the inhospitable seas that lie ahead. . . . The imperative is to launch as many such arks as possible. Some will sink, some will be blown off course, and not all the rest will get through with their cargos intact. But a hopeful spirit, committed to intrinsic good and with faith in surprise, compels us to make the effort. We cannot know the outcome. If we prepare, not for the worst, but for the best, some of our arks will complete their voyage to better days. The more we build, the more will make it.[13]

If we start our ark building today, we might even use the lessons we learn from it to mitigate the damage we are doing to Earth right now, or even reverse it. That next step, however, will require thousands of arks to coalesce into movements that draw their strength from these centers of resilience and change.

Acting Collectively

So often activism is based on what we are against, what we don't
like, what we don't want. And yet we manifest what we focus
on. And so we are manifesting yet ever more of what we don't
want, what we don't like, what we want to change. So for me,
activism is about a spiritual practice as a way of life. And I realized
I didn't climb the tree because I was angry at corporations or the
government, I climbed the tree because when I fell in love with
the redwoods, I fell in love with the world. So it is my
feeling of "connection" that drives me, instead of my
anger and feelings of being disconnected.

—JULIA BUTTERFLY HILL, *THE TAOIST AND THE ACTIVIST*

The battered blue truck slowed and rattled to a stop at a desolate curve
in the road. From my vantage point in the front passenger seat, a
position bestowed on me so I might avoid car sickness on the twisty
roads, the roadside stop was indistinguishable from any other we had
passed in the last half-hour. My companion, Dr. Juan Manuel Canales, leaned forward from the back seat and pointed to a barely visible
opening into the jungle, a few feet up the hillside where the grassy
berm gave way to a tangle of forest. "Un poco mas allá, cien metros
mas o menos en este sendero, vas a ver la entrada, alguien te espera

allí," he said—Someone will meet you if you just go down that narrow trail a few hundred feet. I disembarked, trusting Juan Manuel completely. The driver gave assurances that he'd return to the same spot in a few hours and then quickly continued on his way so as not to draw attention to the stop. Juan Manuel had another community to visit that day, while I was headed to the Zapatista autonomous community of Moises Gandhi. My purpose was to accompany local health promoters and others in deepening our knowledge about pregnancy and childbirth.

It was the late 1990s, a few years after the rebellion began, but the market for Zapatourismo was still going strong. Photogenic Zapatistas in their black ski masks and colorful huipil blouses had captured the imagination of the world. Political tourists from Europe and the United States descended on the Chiapas capital, San Cristobal de las Casas, hoping for a taste of revolution. Many wanted to visit the Autonomous Zone, but access was strictly controlled. The closest most got were the creatively named dishes at the Tierra Adentro Café, like the Omelette Justica or the Huevos Esperanza, or the Zapatista-themed crafts available in the street markets—balaclava-clad dolls and T-shirts depicting Our Lady of Guadalupe in rebel garb.

I had come to Chiapas as a volunteer for Doctors for Global Health, a solidarity group that worked with marginalized and oppressed peoples and saw its role as accompanying the struggle for health and well-being rather than bestowing medical services. Juan Manuel had been recently hired by the organization to work at San Carlos Hospital in Altamirano and provide assistance as requested by neighboring communities. The Zapatistas were deep into their project of forming a self-governing region, eschewing any dependence on or relationship with the Mexican state. Communities in the Zapatista region were under constant threat of infiltration from the Mexican military and paramilitary groups trying to undermine their efforts. For this reason, they were mostly closed to the outside world, although some carefully vetted allies were allowed to participate and support the project. Juan

Manuel, a Mexican physician and activist who had previously worked in the war zones of El Salvador in the 1980s, quickly gained their trust with his humble and patient demeanor.

Like the tourists roaming the markets of San Cristobal, my imagination had been captured by the Zapatistas too. I wanted to learn more about the new world they were building, as well as the courage and vision that made their resistance possible. In the last year of my family medicine residency in Santa Fe, I sought out the mentorship of Charlie Clements, a physician who has dedicated his life to human rights work. Charlie wrote a memoir, *Witness to War*, about his experience in the 1980s when he decided to leave his family medicine residency, travel to El Salvador, and offer his services in rebel-controlled areas during the civil war.[1] I asked Charlie how I could contribute to the efforts of those struggling for justice across the globe, and he told me of his friend from El Salvador days, Juan Manuel, who had just moved to Chiapas to support the Zapatista movement. Although I was certainly young and idealistic, I had a bit more grounding than many of the others drawn to the uprising. Thanks to my Chilean friends, my Spanish was good and I had no delusions about what an oppressive government was capable of doing to squash dissent.

I spent most of my time in Altamirano seeing patients in clinic and covering nighttime call shifts. The hospital was famous for treating combatants from both sides during the uprising. For most of January 1994, the beds were full of injured Indigenous rebels and Mexican soldiers lying side by side in the open wards. To this day, the hospital is one of few places where Indigenous people and those living in the autonomous communities can get essential elements of Western medical care, like surgeries or antibiotics. The nuns who run the place have continued to express solidarity with the Tzeltal, Tojolabal, Tzotzil, Chol, Zoque, Mam, and others who identify with the Zapatistas by providing free care to everyone. Those aligned with the Zapatista movement refuse to accept any aid from the Mexican government, directly or indirectly, so the Sisters were assiduous about rejecting all funding and materials from government sources.

My rare direct contact with the Zapatista communities was mediated through Juan Manuel, who would receive requests for support from local groups and connect appropriate volunteers. On occasion, we'd be invited to participate in classes with health promoters and community health workers co-taught by local leaders and translated from Spanish into local Indigenous languages. The cooperative learning sessions integrated Western medicine with centuries-old healing traditions and midwifery knowledge held by community members.

To understand what inspired the Zapatistas in their extraordinary project of seceding from Mexico and reclaiming and recreating their own nation, one has to go back hundreds of years. From the first contact with the Spanish in the early sixteenth century, Chiapas has been among the most exploited states in Mexico and also among the most resistant to colonial dominance. When Hernan Cortez sent the first Spanish agent to collect taxes and subdue the Indigenous population in 1522, he was fiercely opposed for years. The skirmishes between colonizers and local peoples finally culminated in the Battle of Tepetchia, where many Tzotzils chose suicide by jumping into the steep Cañon del Sumidero over the prospect of submitting to malicious rule by Spanish overlords.[2] In the years that followed, the Spanish and later the Mexicans created a system of haciendas, much like the plantations of the American South—large landholdings and farms made profitable only by forcing Indigenous peoples into lives of slavery and indentured servitude.

Centuries of being enslaved and exploited, of watching their lands deforested and destroyed by wealthy Spanish and Mexican men, and of seeing their peaceful demands for land reform denied, led the native people of Chiapas to devise a revolutionary strategy to take back their homelands in the 1980s. "After 10 years of clandestine organizing in the mountains and jungles of Chiapas, recruiting Indigenous peasants into their guerrilla army and civilian support base, the Zapatistas came to a consensus that they would rather risk dying from a bullet than continue watching their children die from preventable diseases,"[3] wrote Hilary Klein, who spent several years working with Zapatista women's collectives in Chiapas.

The Zapatistas surprised the whole world on that first dawn of 1994 when they rose up and briefly took over much of the state of Chiapas, including San Cristobal de las Casas. Although their initial goal of instigating a revolution and overthrowing the Mexican government fell short, they succeeded in reclaiming over a million acres of their ancestral lands.[4] Ever since that day, they have been fiercely defending their right to create a society organized along their own ideas and principles.

Directly after the uprising, the Zapatista communities asserted their sovereignty and began constructing their own form of self-government. The Autonomous Municipalities were built on long-held cultural values like connection to the land, cooperation, sharing of resources, and reciprocal aid. "Within the Zapatista villages themselves, the deep social fabric of community and the unquestioned assumption that the collective well-being takes priority over the individual, form one of the strongest foundations of the Zapatista movement," Klein writes.[5] They created systems of education, healthcare, justice, communication, and a cooperative economy that employs hundreds of teachers, healers, farmers, artisans, and other workers. Everything starts with the deliberations of hundreds of small assemblies consisting of representatives from a few hundred local families. These community groups of families work to reach decisions by consensus as frequently as possible, then come together with other assemblies in the region to form larger Autonomous Municipalities. In this bottom-up fashion, the Zapatistas' project to retake and rebuild their own educational, healthcare, and economic systems from scratch has been making marked progress for the past three decades.

A full generation after they took up arms, the area under Zapatista control boasts hundreds of schools with thousands of teachers educating children in local languages, culture, and history. The schools follow an egalitarian model of democratic education with curricula decided at the local level. There are many Zapatista-run clinics throughout the region and legions of trained midwives, healers, and community health workers. By many measures, the health status of those living in Zapatista communities has improved and is likely better than those living in neighboring towns outside the Autonomous Zones. Private ownership of land was abolished, and agricultural workers' cooperatives were established using regenerative practices based on Indigenous knowledge on hundreds of farms producing beans, coffee, bananas, sugar, and livestock. Other cooperatives produce textiles, goods for local use, and crafts for export. The Zapatistas have prioritized ecological restoration of their degraded lands, including reforestation projects to protect endangered water sources, while also resisting attempts of outsiders to encroach on their territory for mining and extraction of natural resources like oil and gas.

Everyone in the community, young and old, is engaged in the collective work of creating this new way of life on some level. I experienced this viscerally in the time I spent at Moises Gandhi many years ago. The classes on prenatal care and birth I attended were organized much differently from anything I was used to from my previous educational experiences. Everyone was both teacher and learner, including those with lived experience of pregnancy, traditional midwives from the community, and even the visiting white doctor fresh out of residency. No one was on a pedestal above any other as we practiced listening to fetal heartbeats and discussed different techniques to bring babies safely into this world.

Even as their revolutionary project evolved throughout the years, the Zapatista communities have had to defend their autonomy constantly and continue to suffer frequent threats and violence from both the Mexican government and paramilitary groups representing large ranchers and wealthy landholders. This despite the fact that the Mexican government initially recognized Zapatista sovereignty by agreeing to and signing the San Andres Accords in 1996, recognizing the rights of Indigenous people throughout the nation. The government later reneged on the agreement and instead began a campaign of military harassment of Indigenous peoples that has ebbed and flowed in intensity ever since.

Despite the risks, the number of Autonomous Municipalities has grown over the years with a significant expansion most recently announced in 2019. The area under control now consists of almost half the state. The project was contagious. Other poor and oppressed peoples in the region saw the example of self-government and wanted to participate in the experiment themselves. Although Chiapas is still the poorest state in Mexico and the Indigenous communities continue to endure extreme hardships, the people there express how things have changed since the rebellion began. In 2018 a young Tzotzil spokesperson for the Zapatistas told a *Guardian* reporter, "I am too young to know 1994 but the difference between then and now is that the older generation then did not know if we could even exist [as a people]. Today we have an identity." Another said, "We were forgotten. Now we are known by everyone. In 1994, we had no hospitals or schools. Now we have them. Our work was hard. Now it is much better."[6]

The Indigenous communities' deep connection with the land, despite centuries of concerted efforts to disintegrate that bond and disrupt their culture, led to their drastic decision to take up arms in 1994. The fact that the risk of inaction had become so much greater than the risk of taking action is reflected in the main slogan of the uprising: "Ya Basta!" (Enough Is Enough!). But the Zapatistas required much more than desperation to keep a revolution going for nearly three decades. They have had to employ their fiercest imagination, along with the heartfelt belief that they could create another world, one based around collective flourishing of their own communities, their other-than-human kin, and their whole ecosystems. In the face of continued repression and violence, the Zapatistas are working to carve out a new way of living that could give us all inspiration for the future. Their example continues to reverberate throughout the globe, inspiring many other political movements. Omar Garcia, a leader of the Mexican student uprisings of the past decade, expressed it this way: "The most powerful reference point for us, in terms of knowing that it is possible to change things at their root, are the Zapatista compañeros and their autonomous municipalities."[7]

The Zapatistas are building their own kind of ark, a different way of living on Earth, and they are inviting us all to use their experiment as fodder for our own hopes for the future. What if we dared to follow their example, if we decided that enough was enough, if we refused to see the world through the lens of capitalism and colonialism that has been handed down to us? What if we tried on some new, differently colored glasses? What if we started deeply questioning the hierarchies that divide and disempower us and began imagining new ways of relating to each other and Earth?

Author and activist adrienne maree brown talks about this challenge to our creativity in her book *Emergent Strategy*. We create our own worlds. The concepts of borders and white supremacy, the exaggerated fears of twelve-year-old Black children with toy guns, the ability to call those protecting their ancestral lands "terrorists," and even the idea of capitalism itself, all sprang from human imagination. We can just as easily imagine another world. "We are in an imagination battle," brown writes. "It is so important we fight for our future, get into the game, get dirty, get experimental. How do we create and proliferate a compelling vision of economies and ecologies that center humans and the natural world over the accumulation of material? We embody. We learn . . . but first we imagine."[8]

If we open our eyes and really look around us, we will see many large and small examples of these radical experiments, the hard work of imagining and building new worlds. More frequently than not, the movements are led by Indigenous peoples or others firmly rooted in their homelands and drawing from non-Western cultural traditions.

There are many reasons that deep relationships with land and community are the soil from which so many social movements sprout. We fight for what we love, for our family and kin, with a different kind of passion and intensity than we fight for abstract causes like preventing climate change. Sustaining passion and intensity over time can be tough, so people engaged in the hard work of showing the rest of us how to see the world differently need centers of resilience and safe places to rest and recharge during long and dangerous struggles. Community can provide that place of respite. Finally, the work is too complex and all-encompassing to entrust to just a few charismatic leaders. It requires the combined talents, skills, and creativity of those from many walks of life, and a collective and cooperative mindset.

The struggle against the Dakota Access Pipeline (#NoDAPL) is another dramatic example of a larger political movement emerging from a community-rooted local beginning. The action was started when local youth activists from the Standing Rock Indian Reservation established a camp near the route of the proposed pipeline with the intention of conducting direct actions, asserting their Indigenous sovereignty, and drawing attention to the precious natural and cultural resources endangered by the pipeline. That first camp quickly proliferated into many, as thousands of allies were attracted to the place-based, spontaneous, and collective example of how we might protect the earth and create new worlds. Importantly, those who first gathered at Standing Rock didn't call themselves protesters or activists but rather "water protectors," emphasizing their positive connection to the land and what they were fighting to preserve rather than what they were against. They were fighting to defend what they love, their human and more-than-human kin, and the water their lives literally depend on.

Lakota scholar and activist Nick Estes wrote about the experience of participating in the Standing Rock Oceti Sakowin Camp:

> [There] is something to be learned from the treaty camps at the confluence of the Missouri and Cannonball Rivers. Free food, free education, free health care, free legal aid, a strong sense of community, safety and security were guaranteed to all. Most reservations in the United States don't have access to these services, nor do most poor people. . . . Capitalism is not merely an economic system but also a social system. And it was here abundantly evident that Indigenous social systems offered a radically different way of relating to other people and the world.[9]

In the United States, this kind of decentralized organizing, dependent on deep relationships with community and connection to the land, is not the predominant model we hear about. More often, stories of social change are built on the mythology of individual, charismatic leaders. Even today, most of those political leaders we call "progressive," who voice concern about the consequences of climate change, don't often dare their constituents to envision whole new paradigms or massive collective upheavals. Rather, they urge us to nibble around the edges and be content to get involved on a more individual level—by voting, or writing letters, or contributing money to campaigns or nonprofit organizations. Many of us engage in those actions and feel as if we have done all we can. We are limited by the stories that those in power want us to believe, but we can create other stories for ourselves, just as the Zapatistas have done.

Radical change can feel scary. We get comfortable with the familiar, even with our dissatisfaction. We imagine that wars or natural disasters or violence or pollution won't ever reach our neighborhood. In the United States, fully 72 percent of us believe that global warming is happening and about 70 percent agree that it will harm plants and animals, future generations, and people in developing countries, but only 47 percent, a minority, think that it will harm them personally.[10] As the effects of climate change become more and more undeniable, a significant number of our neighbors find themselves ever more firmly mired in denial. The future seems so ominous and inevitable, it's easy to see how a sense of powerlessness can become overwhelming when the work ahead is so daunting. But being "radical" doesn't have to be alarming. Activist and author Angela Davis pointed out that the word *radical* "just means grasping things at the root." To find those roots, we must become more solidly rooted ourselves.

In these pages, I've invited the reader to imagine different narratives and to hear stories about alternative ways of living that are endangered or even extinct. It's part love letter to the almost-forgotten past of our species, and part beacon to a possible hopeful future. I started off by pointing out what should be obvious to us all, that we are embedded in ecosystems, in communities of other beings, whether we are aware of it or not. The writer David Foster Wallace opened his famous commencement speech with a story of an elder fish swimming by and greeting two younger fishes. The old fish says, "Morning, boys. How's the water?" The two young fish swim on for a bit, and then eventually one of them looks over at the other and goes "What the hell is water?" We get caught up in the rhythms and needs of our everyday lives, our routes from home to work or school and back again, our basic needs for shelter and food and diversion. We walk around with blinders on and fail to see the possibilities of different worlds. There is a great dance whirling all around us. We can make the choice to see it, to fall in love with it, and to join in with our own choreography.

Once we start looking for community, we will see it everywhere, along with many opportunities to jump in and start dancing. It just takes a few of us to start showing another way and it catches on like wildfire. Look around your local community and I guarantee you will find those already engaged in building arks, in creating new worlds and different ways of seeing.

In my own community, I look to the example of Tewa Women United and the Healing Oasis Garden they created, or to groups like Amigos Bravos, a New Mexico organization that helps strengthen the ability of communities to value and preserve their own waterways and acequia systems. Twenty years ago, few of us had any idea what the word *fracking* meant. By 2010, the Community Environmental Legal Defense Fund helped activists in Pittsburgh pass the first-ever local fracking ban in the nation. Since then, over 400 localities have passed ordinances to ban or restrict fracking, including the states of Vermont, Maryland, Oregon and Washington.[11] Being a new dancer means following the lead of others, learning the steps of those who came before you, but also adding in your particular style and flair. We can find much inspiration in the cooperative and communal ways of the natural world.

Adrienne maree brown looks to the examples of migrating birds and writes, "There is an art to flocking: staying separate enough not to crowd each other, aligned enough to maintain a shared direction, and cohesive enough to always move towards each other."[12] I think this drive to connect and cooperate and dance together is inherent in us, even stronger than our need to compete and achieve and get on top. Birds don't need to be taught the art of murmuration; they just need to be reminded of what they already know in their bones. Once we feel what it's like to live in community, to know that we are supported and not alone, to care for our neighbors of all species, we immediately understand that this is how we are intended to live. We're just out of practice.

The premise of this book is that what is good for the earth is also good for our personal and collective well-being as *Homo sapiens*, and this is also true of the act of joining together in communal action. I have described how connections to community and nature can improve health. Having a shared vision and goal just amplifies the effect. A sample of over 13,000 older adults in the US assessed over a period of eight years showed that those who maintained their sense of purpose over time were more likely to stay physically active and maintain a healthy weight.[13] Worrying about the world's problems didn't keep them up at night, either. They were 33 percent less likely to develop sleep problems as well.

Our world is divided. Millions of people find themselves in the same predicament as the Zapatistas; the risk of continuing down the same path has become intolerable. Millions more convince themselves they are not in such dire straits, that their wealth and privilege will shield them from the most unpleasant effects of the world we've created. But what of their children, and what of the whole world? What of those life-sustaining ecosystems that every one of us, rich and poor, requires for survival? Gaia herself is on the brink.

Wherever we find ourselves in that continuum, we are all floating along in that same toxic river. Some of us have boats, some have rickety rafts, and some are swimming in the muck. Most of the efforts to keep us from harm are centered on fixing a few leaky boats or offering swimming lessons. The Zapatistas got sick of the lessons. They already knew how to swim, or they would've drowned centuries ago. They were tired of the same international aid organizations showing them how to form craft cooperatives or offering fragmented healthcare programs targeted at a single disease. The only real solution they could see was to clean up the whole river at the source. It doesn't happen overnight. It takes decades of organizing, of relationship building, of remembering and amplifying our ancestors' stories.

Never in the history of the world was a problem solved without first imagining a solution, a better way. To the stark challenges that face humanity right now—our warming planet, diminishing biodiversity, vanishing wild places, and worsening human health—there is not one answer. We won't be saved by a single solution. We need a million solutions rising up from a million collective imaginations and a million centers of resilience and experimentation, all of them taking on the big questions: How can we live differently on the earth? How might we let go of competition and instead harness the power of collaboration with all living things? How can we remember our old nurturing place in our ecosystems? The answers to those questions will show us how to build the kinds of arks we need to get through the storms and floods ahead. What has been laid out in these pages in just one possible roadmap, one path to that imagined future. Being open to all these ideas, all these experiments rising up from thousands of places, is the only way to salvation.

Epilogue
The Coyote and
the Cottonwood

All that you touch
You Change.
All that you Change
Changes you.
The only lasting truth
Is Change.
God
Is Change.

—*Octavia Butler, Parable of the Sower*

When I started writing this book, I didn't know where it would lead, I just knew I was frustrated, and that I spent too many days in the clinic feeling ineffectual. The unspoken promise throughout my medical education was that if I mastered the art of medicine, I'd be able to diagnose and treat most health problems presented to me. That is certainly the assumption many of my patients bring into the exam room. In reality, I felt like I was just nibbling around the edges of the root causes of my patients' maladies. For example, during my medical education I learned the specific diagnostic criteria for depression and the biological basis for and success rates of various antidepressant pills.

In practice, if I took time to listen to the stories behind the diagnosis, each case of "depression" in my patients seemed unique. Some were struggling in violent relationships, some had dire financial woes and were facing eviction, some were dealing with personal losses and overwhelming grief. In cases where societal ills were the root cause, prescribing a pill to the individual in my exam room felt like I was treating the wrong patient.

My medical education was of little help in figuring out what kinds of "prescriptions" could help the *right* patient, but through years of practicing medicine, studying public health, and living as a human on Earth, I came to understand that the answer lay in strengthening our relationships and communities—with humans and all other beings. Humans cannot be healthy when the ecosystems they inhabit are sick and suffering. But how to treat a whole ecosystem? I still don't have all the answers, but through writing this book and exploring ideas of many other writers and thinkers who have come to similar conclusions, I think I can offer some suggestions.

The first step is cultivating and deepening an active awareness that we are all enmeshed in a great web of connections, and that the essential well-being of all living things depends on those connections. The network of life doesn't look anything like a pyramid. There are no hierarchies. Even "survival of the fittest" is a myth. Our survival and health depend much more on cooperation than competition. Modern society sings a siren song of individualism and consumerism, trying to convince us that we need to achieve more, earn more, have more followers, get more stuff in order to feel good, but that's all a ruse. None of those things are important to our well-being. Studies show that "happiness" flatlines after we earn enough to sustainably meet the basic needs of ourselves and our loved ones.[1] So the first prescription is to cultivate a different worldview, shifting focus from self to community, from human-centric to life-centric. Just noticing all the life around us is a good first step, or learning the names of the trees in your yard, or the unique features of the birds who share your neighborhood.

Practicing Kin Awareness

Recently I camped out at Ghost Ranch for a writing retreat, the place made famous by painter Georgia O'Keeffe, who lived there much of her life. It was her querencia. As I set off one morning for a hike in the arroyo, the ravens were involved in their usual morning conversation. RAWK RAWK from one side of the canyon. A pause and then another rhythmic RAWK RAWK in reply.

An array of gnarled junipers looked down on me and I started photographically cataloging them to study later. Some were thriving, some were half dead, some were all the way dead. Some were barely hanging on to the cliff's edge by a few roots. Their twisted shapes enchanted Georgia; she painted one in particular and made it famous. I wondered how she could limit herself. If I were I painter, I could spend a lifetime painting just these, each with its own story to tell.

A boulder bigger than my camper, recently dislodged, nearly blocked my way. It had to have fallen this season because the surface was still caked with thick red mud, a few plants clinging to it, not yet knowing that their days were numbered. The next big storm would flood this gulch and surely wash them away. I passed one stunted cottonwood tree among the juniper and piñon, a broadleaf, with only a few tufts of leaves and one yellowed branch. I wondered if my cottonwood at home had started to turn while I'm here.

My progress was finally stopped where the arroyo gave way to an impassable rocky canyon edge, the site of a temporary waterfall after hard rains. The way back home looked entirely different than the way there, even though it was the same path. I noticed the small things on the arroyo floor on the way back. Lichens impossibly thriving on rocks. They too are tiny communities of different organisms supporting each other in harsh conditions. A sage completely engulfed by a mountain mahogany, a rare happy marriage. The primroses were closed, but their potential was evident. A few hours later, when the sun touches them, they will fully open glorious yellow blossoms. A lone piñon jay flew across my path. I had only ever seen them before in flocks.

As I wrote this back at camp, a rabbit kept a watchful eye. He hopped within twenty feet before noticing me and freezing in place. His ears pulled all the way back as he hunched close to the ground and tried to disappear into shadow, looking annoyed and wary at the same time.

While on my walk, had I experienced a sudden calm, an almost-physical tingling sensation, and felt deeply embedded in the world around me. I remember having this same feeling often when I was a teenager walking in woods with my black lab, a wave of deep love for the world and all the living beings that inhabit it.

The rabbit loosened up after a bit and decided he trusted me enough to nibble on some grasses and turn his back, carrying on with his day. I thought about resilience and what we all need to trust, to thrive, to realize our potential, to bloom completely like the primroses—just a little water and sun.

Cultivating Interdependence

Once we become aware that our very bodies are ecosystems enmeshed in overlapping and concentrically larger ecosystems, we naturally come to understand the importance of cultivating and nourishing the relationships that sustain us. In this endeavor, it helps to observe other creatures in our lives with humility and curiosity, without judgment, and to confront our own prejudices and unfounded fears. As an example, consider the coyote and cottonwood.

Most folks can understand the affection I have for my cottonwood friend. He is majestic and beautiful. Right now he is thriving, but several years ago when he shed most of his branches, there was only a huge gaping hole with a couple of gangly arms on either side. Since then, he has healed and the wound is almost filled with new growth. In summer, the wind rustling through his long limbs sounds like waves breaking on the ocean shore; in fall his backlit mango-yellow leaves glow and dance in spectacular sunset displays. He is gorgeous—what's not to love?

My coyote brethren, on the other hand, are much reviled and feared. I haven't seen Red (the coyote I cured of mange) for a few years now, maybe because I've been less vigilant in keeping up with trail cameras, or maybe because healthy coyotes can hunt for themselves and don't frequent the compost pile so much. On social media, coyote myths are constantly springing up—about their wily ways of luring pet dogs ostensibly to play while leading them into a trap to be attacked by the pack; or their propensity to attack young children, for example. But in eight years of living in this community of many humans and dogs and coyotes, I've yet to hear such a story. To be sure, coyotes have availed themselves of available meals, either from the compost, or the chicken coop, or an outdoor cat who's a little too slow. They are predators, but they are also wary of humans. The Urban Coyote Research Project found that between 1960 and 2006, there were only 142 incidents of coyote attacks on humans, and there have been only two confirmed incidents of coyotes killing humans in North America, this despite upwards of 10 million coyotes living in increasingly closer proximity to hundreds of millions of humans.[2]

Creating real community within the natural world and the human one is only possible if we examine the origins of our biases and learn to see the value in all life. When we listen with empathy to what a tree or an animal or a neighbor shares with us, we build relationships based on common cause and solidarity. By confronting and dismantling our baseless fears, we can create connections and relationships without hierarchies. In the process, we'll fall in love with the world in a whole new way.

Contributing Our Gifts

With awareness that we are all part of ecosystems and with intention to create and deepen relationships from a life-centric point of view, seeing ways we can fit in and contribute comes naturally. In the words of Robin Wall Kimmerer, we can behave as naturalized members of our communities, like the plantains, rather than gentrifiers or colonizers, like the kudzu. Or as Terry Tempest Williams says, "Finding beauty in a broken world is creating beauty in the world we find."[3] When we spend time listening and observing, we start to understand the rhythms, customs, and languages of the places we inhabit, and we can figure out how to swim with the current of our communities and become useful constituents. From this new sense of kinship, we'll know what we can offer and also where to turn when we need to ask for help. The idea of mutual aid is based in the knowledge that we all need support sometimes—today maybe I'm helping you, tomorrow it will be reversed. It's an active acknowledgment of our interdependence.

In my own life, I try to pay attention to those deeply satisfying moments when I feel at home and connected, a part of something larger than myself—the comforting sensation of querencia. I have been lucky to experience that kind of acceptance and interdependence many times—when I was at a peña, or song circle, with my friends in Chile in my twenties, learning to play Spanish folk songs on my guitar and about how they survived the Pinochet years by supporting each other. Or in my thirties, with the Zapatistas, learning that creating a literal whole other world was possible, limited only by our collective imaginations. Or later in my Near West Side community in Cleveland, seeing how simple things like community yoga classes or weekly potluck knitting circles can knit communities together. Or here in New Mexico, coming to understand the centuries of connection between humans and the land unique to this place, and sharing equally in the labor to maintain our valley's own ecosystem during the spring and fall ditch cleanings. All of these are a little taste of what kinds of communities are possible. Like Mr. Rogers implored us, look for the helpers, they will be building the arks, the places of resilience and strength we will need to get through the coming turbulent times.

An Accumulation of Acts

I'm writing these last paragraphs on the cusp between winter and spring—a season that's unpredictable and pregnant with possibility.

On any given day it could snow six inches or be seventy degrees and sunny. When I was younger, my favorite time of year was the fall, back when death and decay seemed like abstract, romantic ideas. As I get closer to the end of my own life, I love this time of year best. It's an in-between space, not quite one season or the other, where surprising things happen and the only constant is change. My friend John has come by to prune the fruit trees, as he does in this season when they are just awakening but before they explode with blossoms. His family has deep roots in New Mexico and he is revitalizing an old, tangled apple orchard on their ancestral homestead up near Taos. We walk through the backyard, pausing to have a conversation with the trees in the orchard.

As we amble down crooked rows, we assess how each tree has come through the past year. A few didn't make it, including my beloved Italian plum and the Orcas Island pear. The plum was an homage to my Italian upbringing and a favorite for pastries. The pear was a nod to my time in the Northwest, especially at a friend's cabin on a remote San Juan Island. "This is very far from Orcas Island," the stunted tree seems to have said, "what did you expect?" I am still learning how to listen to the land and refrain from imposing my own nostalgic ideas. We pause by the quince who is putting on new growth for the first time since I planted him next to the acequia a couple of years ago, the pear who sprang back with redoubled vigor from root stock, the peaches who have been struggling with disease for years and against all odds seem to be flourishing for the first time, and finally the old cherry, maybe in her sunset years, her lower branches dying off, but still with lots of vigor in the uppermost limbs where the magpies take the cherries I can't reach.

We notice other things too. I remark that there are fewer magpies now in the neighborhood than a few years ago, maybe because more ravens have moved in. Stopping at the pond, we peer through the thin film of ice to see if the salamanders have laid eggs yet. John sees a yellow polka-dotted tail flick briefly among last year's submerged gray-green lily pads. I'm glad I mucked out the piles of accumulated sand from the acequia last fall, because somehow, miraculously, almost before the ice clears, the salamanders have returned to lay their eggs, and I wouldn't want to disturb them now with that task. Mysteriously, some have already managed their spring migration through the still snow-covered field, back to the pond where they were born. We don't see eggs today, but in the next few days and for weeks to come, the pond will be overflowing with them, covering every underwater twig and leaf. As we amble through the landscape, we find birth and death, but also inexplicable resilience. Everything feels like it's on the brink of transformation.

The whole world seems suspended right now in this liminal space, a borderland between polarization and connection, war and peace, survival and extinction. All futures are still imaginable, maybe still within reach. Will we choose to find our way back to being a keystone species, or will we continue being a kerosene species, picking and choosing what seems pleasing to us in the moment and destroying everything else? Will the human species turn out to be too smart for its own good? The technologies we've invented are beyond the dreams of our ancestors just a few generations ago, but will we use them for the collective well-being of all, or for the benefit of a few privileged individuals?

There are always glimpses of what the world could be, of cross-species collaborations like news stories about people working for hours to free a beached whale, of communities working together to overcome adversities like wildfires and floods, of people caring for their ecosystems whether it's a windowsill garden or a wildlife refuge. As Clarissa Pinkola Estés says, "It is not given to us to know which acts or by whom, will cause the critical mass to tip toward an enduring good. What is needed for dramatic change is an accumulation of acts—adding, adding to, adding more, continuing. We know that it does not take 'everyone on Earth' to bring justice and peace, but only a small, determined group who will not give up during the first, second, or hundredth gale."[4]

It's my hope that the stories in this book will inspire you to become part of a group that will not give up. By embracing our embeddedness in ecosystems and communities, in the natural and human worlds, and by leveraging all our human creativity, our relationships become networks and finally coalesce into the sweeping social change our dire situation demands. The very process of bringing this book into being would not have been possible without a lifetime of openness to hearing the stories and ideas and experiences of thousands of patients, friends, colleagues, elders, and admired creators and thinkers. If it provides just one stepping stone in the path, and if it inspires others to add their step-stones as well, it will have accomplished its goal. I don't know exactly where the path will take us, but I am certain we can create it together and find the way back to restoring balance and wellness for all.

Author's Note

A few disclaimers and clarifications.

First, the patient stories I've told in the book are all true, from my own clinic, but some details and names have been changed to preserve confidentiality.

Second, a note about pronouns. The reader will notice that I use them, while acknowledging that pronouns are sometimes a trap. In many cases I use gendered pronouns to refer to other-than-human beings including Earth her/their-self. I understand this is not ideal, but alternatives are also problematic. Until new pronouns are invented that convey an equal sense of personhood without adding in gendered stereotypes, options are limited.

Another problematic pronoun is *we*. I have tried to limit its use to only when I intentionally mean "all humankind" or even "all beings" while acknowledging that all humans do not bear equal responsibility for the state of the Earth as it is. I have tried to avoid the too common habit of lazily using the pronoun in a way that generalizes my very specific experience as a white woman living in the United States. When I do use *we*, I have attempted to call all of us "in" and also to appeal to our common sense of solidarity. I hope I have succeeded, but please let me know if I've missed the mark.

Acknowledgments

These days Indigenous land acknowledgments are commonplace. My awareness that the land I live on is occupied territory, taken from the Tewa and Keres peoples by force, is always with me. I have not so often seen Indigenous knowledge acknowledgments. Within the book, I have cited the Indigenous origins of many of the ideas presented, but in reality, the concept for the whole book rests on the vast sum of Indigenous science and philosophy from what is now called North and South America, Asia, Europe, Australia, and Africa. I hope we continue to be curious and learn from the accumulated knowledge of Indigenous people while acknowledging that in many, many cases, Indigenous people thought of it first.

A writer friend says that writing is a team sport, and it certainly has been for me. I have been honored to have the accompaniment of a slew of wonderful writers. From almost the beginning of this journey I've relied on the wisdom of book midwife, coach, and editor Carolyn Flynn. I am deeply indebted to Nassim Assefi for being one of the first champions of this book and encouraging me to apply for the wonderful Hedgebrook women's writing residency. My Hedgebrook cohort of Jael Humphrey, Heidi Durrow, Diana Xin, Roja Heydarpour, Julie Phillips, and Michelle Ruiz Keil continue to be inspirational writing mentors, mutual fan club, and support group all rolled into one. I'm also grateful to all the folks at Mesa Refuge Residency for accepting me into their community and especially to Vanessa Daniel and Tara Duggan, my Point Reyes housemates, for their friendship and encouragement.

Many thanks to Teju Cole for his generosity in offering mentorship to essential workers who are also writers and photographers during the height of the pandemic. His excellent and thoughtful playlists have been the soundtrack that fueled much of my writing.

Thank you also to:

Enrique Salmon, Dan Pink, Juan Manuel Canales, Raj Patel, George Trujillo, and William deBuys for their gifts of time and attention.

Kira Jones, Jessica Smyser, Erin Elder, Hallelujah Strongheart, and Hez Aronson for their early support and feedback.

Readers who helped improve the manuscript with their sharp eyes and insightful comments, especially David Martin of Middle Creek Publishing; Louella Bryant; Sonora Jha and my colleagues in Hugo House's book lab, Ariel Ayers, CT Moon, Hira Bluestone, Hera McCloud and Amelia Schmidt; and Scott Wolven and Shanna McNair of The Writer's Hotel.

The talented staff of North Atlantic Books, especially Tim McKee and Gillian Hamel. I'm so happy we found each other and I can't imagine a better home for this book.

Many people offered encouragement and support along the way, never doubting I could accomplish what at times seemed impossible. They include Molly Wieser, Sarah Knopp, Robin McLean, Dona Bolding, Amy Hanauer, Earl Pike, Roshi Joan Halifax, Lesley Poling-Kempes, Kyra Ryan Ochoa, Joshua Billiter, Michelle Bates, Melissa Howden, Dan Smith, Darrin Ehardt, Cecile Lipworth, Stephanie Tade, all the Flying Flounders, and the folks at the Lannan Foundation, among many others.

Deep gratitude to the late Dr. Paul Farmer, who had faith in me and this book and helped bring it to light. I am one of thousands of health workers who continue to be inspired by his life and work and frequently invoke the mantra "What would Paul do?"

• • •

Thank you to all my ancestors who held much of this knowledge and lived close to the land, in the Alps of northern Italy, on the shores of the Adriatic, and in the forests of southern Sweden. I hope I have unearthed some of the genetic wisdom you bestowed on me.

● ● ●

Finally, none of this would be possible without the loving upbringing I had thanks to my parents, Mary and Bruce Johnson. They instilled in me my love of nature, spirit of generosity and community, and sense of fairness and equity. Thank you, Mom and Dad.

Notes

Introduction: Out of the Fire

1 Simon Romero, "The Government Set a Colossal Wildfire. What Are Victims Owed?," *New York Times*, June 21, 2022, www.nytimes.com/2022/06/21/us/new-mexico-wildfire-forest-service.html.

2 Phaedra Haywood, "Mora Residents File Lawsuit over Fire Information," *Santa Fe New Mexican*, July 15, 2023, www.santafenewmexican.com/news/local_news/mora-residents-file-lawsuit-over-fire-information/article_473de796-e812-11ec-97f6-a332b87f16ac.html.

3 Dan McKay, "New Mexico's Largest Wildfire: Devastation Lingers One Year Since Spark That Lit Hermits Peak Blaze," *Albuquerque Journal*, June 7, 2023, www.abqjournal.com/news/local/new-mexicos-largest-wildfire-devastation-lingers-one-year-since-spark-that-lit-hermits-peak-blaze/article_e2931305-1d6a-5959-ad82-23824784207e.html.

4 Simon Romero, "'Burning Down a Way of Life': Wildfire Rips Through a Hispanic Bastion," *New York Times*, May 5, 2022, www.nytimes.com/2022/05/05/us/new-mexico-wildfires.html.

5 Timothy Morton, *The Ecological Thought* (Harvard University Press, 2010).

6 Lynn Margulis, *Symbiotic Planet: A New Look at Evolution* (Basic Books, 1998).

Chapter 1. The Wild Tithe

1 Gary Snyder, *The Practice of the Wild: Essays* (North Point, 1990), 36.

2 Michelle Nijhuis, "After Bears Ears and Grand Staircase-Escalante, Where Will Trump's War on Public Lands End?," *New Yorker*, December 6, 2017.

3 Robin Wall Kimmerer, *Braiding Sweetgrass* (Milkweed Editions, 2014), 5.

Chapter 2: The Mess We're In

1 Frank Edwards, Lee Hedwig, and Michael H. Esposito, "Risk of Being Killed by Police Use of Force in the United States by Age, Race-Ethnicity, and Sex," *Proceedings of the National Academy of Sciences* 116, no. 34 (August 5, 2019): 16793–98, https://doi.org/10.31235/osf.io/kw9cu.

2 Christopher Ingram, "How Rising Inequality Hurts Everyone, Even the Rich," *Washington Post*, February 6, 2018, www.washingtonpost.com/news /wonk/wp/2018/02/06/how-rising-inequality-hurts-everyone-even -the-rich.

3 Hannah Ritchie, Veronika Samborska, and Max Roser, "Urbanization," Our World in Data, February 23, 2024, https://ourworldindata.org /urbanization.

4 William Park, "How City Life Affects Your Health and Happiness," BBC News, February 24, 2022, www.bbc.com/future/article/20190816-is-city -life-really-bad-for-you.

5 Meng Wang et al., "Association Between Long-Term Exposure to Ambient Air Pollution and Change in Quantitatively Assessed Emphysema and Lung Function," *JAMA* 322, no. 6 (August 13, 2019): 546, https://doi.org /10.1001/jama.2019.10255.

6 Michael Brauer, "State of Global Air 2024," Institute for Health Metrics and Evaluation, June 19, 2024, www.healthdata.org/research-analysis/library /state-global-air-2024.

7 Kathleen Magramo, "A Third of Pakistan Is Underwater amid Its Worst Floods in History," CNN, September 2, 2022, www.cnn.com/2022/09/02 /asia/pakistan-floods-climate-explainer-intl-hnk/index.html.

8 Nouran Salahieh, Jason Hanna, and Amir Vera, "Jackson, Mississippi, Residents Told to Shower with Mouths Closed as Water Treatment Plant Repairs Continue on Day 4 of Water Shortage," CNN, September 2, 2022, www.cnn.com/2022/09/01/us/jackson-water-system-failing-thursday /index.html.

9 "Libya: Slow Flood Recovery Failing Displaced Survivors," Human Rights Watch, September 10, 2024, www.hrw.org/news/2024/09/10/libya-slow -flood-recovery-failing-displaced-survivors.

10 Andrew D. Hwang, "7.5 Billion and Counting: How Many Humans Can the Earth Support?," The Conversation, July 9, 2018, https://theconversation .com/7-5-billion-and-counting-how-many-humans-can-the-earth-support -98797.

11 "Facts About the Nature Crisis," UNEP, 2022, www.unep.org/facts-about -nature-crisis.

12 "Chart: Globally, 70% of Freshwater Is Used for Agriculture," *Data Blog*, World Bank, March 22, 2017, https://blogs.worldbank.org/en/opendata /chart-globally-70-freshwater-used-agriculture.

13 Elizabeth Kolbert, *The Sixth Extinction: An Unnatural History* (Picador, 2014), 16.

14 R. E. A. Almond, M. Grooten, D. Juffe Bignoli, and T. Petersen, eds., *Living Planet Report 2022: Building a Nature-Positive Society*, World Wildlife Fund, 2022, www.wwf.org.uk/sites/default/files/2023-05/WWF-Living-Planet -Report-2022.pdf.

15 David Wallace-Wells, *The Uninhabitable Earth: Life After Warming* (Penguin Random House, 2019).

Chapter 3: How Did We Get Here?

1 Paul Bauer, "Geology of the Taos Area: Geologic History," Astronaut Geophysical Training, NASA/New Mexico Bureau of Geology and Mineral Resources, 1999, https://geoinfo.nmt.edu/geoscience/projects/astronauts /geologic_history.html.

2 Sondra Jones, *Being and Becoming Ute: The Story of an American Indian People* (University of Utah Press, 2019), 14.

3 Jones, *Being and Becoming Ute*, 50–51.

4 "Southern Ute Indian Tribe: History," Southern Ute Indian Tribe, 2024, www.southernute-nsn.gov/history.

5 Jones, *Being and Becoming Ute*, 49.

6 Nick Johnson, ed., "Treaty of Abiquiú," Colorado Encyclopedia, n.d., accessed August 28, 2024, https://coloradoencyclopedia.org/article/treaty -abiquiu.

7 James A. Crutchfield, Candy Moulton, and Terry A. Del Bene, *The Settlement of America: Encyclopedia of Westward Expansion from Jamestown to the Closing of the Frontier* (Routledge, 2015), 161–62.

8 Christopher Ketcham, "The Rogue Agency," *Harper's*, March 2016.

9 David Graeber and David Wengrow, *The Dawn of Everything: A New History of Humanity* (Picador/Farrar, Straus and Giroux, 2023), 463–68.

10 Charles C. Mann, *1491: New Revelations of the Americas Before Columbus* (Vintage, 2011), 50.

11 "Interview with Wade Davis: On the Edge, Timbuktu," *Radio Expeditions*, NPR, May 27, 2003, https://legacy.npr.org/programs/re/archivesdate/2003 /may/mali/davisinterview.html.

12 Yuval N. Harari, *Sapiens: A Brief History of Humankind* (Harper Perennial, 2018), 212.

13 Thomas W. Merrill, "Masters and Possessors of Nature," *The New Atlantis*, September 26, 2020, www.thenewatlantis.com/publications/masters-and -possessors-of-nature.

14 Aristotle, *Politics* (Clarendon Press, 1905).

15 "Scientific Racism," Harvard Library, 2024, https://library.harvard.edu
    /confronting-anti-black-racism/scientific-racism.
16 Keith Bradley, "Animalizing the Slave: The Truth of Fiction," *Journal of
    Roman Studies* 90 (November 2000): 110–25, https://doi.org/10.2307
    /300203.
17 Frederick Douglass, *Narrative of the Life of Frederick Douglass, an American
    Slave* (Anti-Slavery Office, 1849), 45.
18 "Doctrine of Discovery," Upstander Project, 2024, https://upstanderproject
    .org/learn/guides-and-resources/first-light/doctrine-of-discovery.
19 Matthew Wood, "Harvey and the Witches: RCP Museum," Royal College
    of Physicians Museum, April 18, 2018, https://history.rcplondon.ac.uk/blog
    /harvey-and-witches.

Chapter 4. Gardens or Machines

 1 Dhruv Khullar, "Do You Trust the Medical Profession?," *New York Times*,
    January 23, 2018.
 2 "Bill of the Month," NPR, accessed August 28, 2024, www.npr.org/series
    /651784144/bill-of-the-month.
 3 Naykky Singh Ospina et al., "Eliciting the Patient's Agenda: Secondary
    Analysis of Recorded Clinical Encounters," *Journal of General Internal Medicine*
    34, no. 1 (July 2, 2018): 36–40, https://doi.org/10.1007/s11606-018
    -4540-5.
 4 Ben Roitberg, "Tyranny of a 'Randomized Controlled Trials,'" *Surgical
    Neurology International* 3, no. 1 (2012): 154, https://doi.org/10.4103/2152
    -7806.104748.
 5 Rebecca A. Clay, "The Pitfalls of Randomized Controlled Trials," *Monitor
    on Psychology*, September 2010, www.apa.org/monitor/2010/09/trials.
 6 Brian Resnick, "The Weird Power of the Placebo Effect, Explained," Vox,
    July 7, 2017, www.vox.com/science-and-health/2017/7/7/15792188
    /placebo-effect-explained.
 7 Barbara Ehrenreich and Deirdre English, *Witches, Midwives, and Nurses: A
    History of Women Healers* (Feminist Press at the City University of New
    York, 2010), 86–87.
 8 Arthur Boylston, "The Origins of Inoculation," *Journal of the Royal Society of
    Medicine* 105, no. 7 (July 2012): 309–13, https://doi.org/10.1258/jrsm
    .2012.12k044.
 9 René Descartes, *Meditations on First Philosophy: With Selections from the
    Objections and Replies*, trans. John Cottingham (Cambridge University
    Press, 2017).

10 Lara C. Kovell et al., "US Hypertension Management Guidelines: A Review of the Recent Past and Recommendations for the Future," *Journal of the American Heart Association* 4, no. 12 (December 2015), https://doi .org/10.1161/jaha.115.002315.

11 Hunter K. Holt et al., "Differences in Hypertension Medication Prescribing for Black Americans and Their Association with Hypertension Outcomes," *Journal of the American Board of Family Medicine* 35, no. 1 (January 2022): 26–34, https://doi.org/10.3122/jabfm.2022.01.210276.

12 Kelly M. Hoffman et al., "Racial Bias in Pain Assessment and Treatment Recommendations, and False Beliefs About Biological Differences Between Blacks and Whites," *Proceedings of the National Academy of Sciences* 113, no. 16 (April 4, 2016): 4296–4301, https://doi.org/10.1073 /pnas.1516047113.

13 James A. Diao and Adewole S. Adamson, "Representation and Misdiagnosis of Dark Skin in a Large-Scale Visual Diagnostic Challenge," *Journal of the American Academy of Dermatology* 86, no. 4 (April 2022): 950–51, https://doi.org/10.1016/j.jaad.2021.03.088; K. Shao and H. Feng, "Racial and Ethnic Healthcare Disparities in Skin Cancer in the United States: A Review of Existing Inequities, Contributing Factors, and Potential Solutions," *Journal of Clinical and Aesthetic Dermatology* 15, no. 7 (July 2022): 16–22.

14 "What Is a Community Health Center?," NACHC, January 11, 2024, www.nachc.org/community-health-centers/what-is-a-health-center.

15 Judy Schader Rogers, *Out in the Rural*, 1970, https://www.youtube.com /watch?v=944DNLy1nHQ.

16 Denise Grady, "H. Jack Geiger, Doctor Who Fought Social Ills, Dies at 95," *New York Times*, December 28, 2020.

Chapter 5. Our Bodies Are Ecosystems

1 Kenneth Joseph Arrow, Claire Panosian, and Hellen Gelband, *Saving Lives, Buying Time: Economics of Malaria Drugs in an Age of Resistance* (National Academies Press, 2004).

2 J. David Hacker, "Decennial Life Tables for the White Population of the United States, 1790–1900," *Historical Methods* 43, no. 2 (April 30, 2010): 45–79, https://doi.org/10.1080/01615441003720449.

3 "Health History: Health and Longevity Since the Mid-19th Century," Stanford University School of Medicine, January 2, 2023, https://geriatrics .stanford.edu/ethnomed/african_american/fund/health_history/longevity .html.

4 Michael Haines, "Fertility and Mortality in the United States," Economic History Association, March 19, 2008, https://eh.net/encyclopedia/fertility -and-mortality-in-the-united-states.

5 "NIH Human Microbiome Project Defines Normal Bacterial Makeup of the Body," National Institutes of Health, August 31, 2015, www.nih.gov /news-events/news-releases/nih-human-microbiome-project-defines-normal -bacterial-makeup-body.

6 Scott F. Gilbert and Alfred I. Tauber, "Rethinking Individuality: The Dialectics of the Holobiont," *Biology & Philosophy* 31, no. 6 (October 19, 2016): 839–53, https://doi.org/10.1007/s10539-016-9541-3.

7 Gary Paul Nabhan, *Food, Genes, and Culture: Eating Right for Your Origins* (Island Press, 2013), 1.

8 Vinod K. Gupta, Sandip Paul, and Chitra Dutta, "Geography, Ethnicity or Subsistence-Specific Variations in Human Microbiome Composition and Diversity," *Frontiers in Microbiology* 8 (June 23, 2017), https://doi.org /10.3389/fmicb.2017.01162.

9 Daniel Ren Yap et al., "Beyond a Vestigial Organ: Effects of the Appendix on Gut Microbiome and Colorectal Cancer," *Journal of Gastroenterology and Hepatology* 39, no. 5 (February 2024): 826–35, https://doi.org/10.1111 /jgh.16497.

10 Evan M. Holbrook et al., "Mycobacterium Vaccae NCTC 11659, a Soil-Derived Bacterium with Stress Resilience Properties, Modulates the Proinflammatory Effects of LPS in Macrophages," *International Journal of Molecular Sciences* 24, no. 6 (March 8, 2023): 5176, https://doi.org/10.3390 /ijms24065176.

Chapter 6. Gaia's Biome

1 "Federal Judge Strikes Down 'Lake Erie Bill of Rights,'" Animal Legal Defense Fund, April 3, 2024, https://aldf.org/article/federal-judge-strikes -down-lake-erie-bill-of-rights.

2 Gwendolyn Gordon, "Environmental Personhood," SSRN, 2017, https:// doi.org/10.2139/ssrn.2935007.

3 Tiffany Challe, "The Rights of Nature—Can an Ecosystem Bear Legal Rights?," State of the Planet, Columbia Climate School, April 22, 2021, https://news.climate.columbia.edu/2021/04/22/rights-of-nature -lawsuits.

4 Anna V. Smith, "The Klamath River Now Has the Legal Rights of a Person," *High Country News*, September 24, 2019, www.hcn.org/issues/51.18/tribal -affairs-the-klamath-river-now-has-the-legal-rights-of-a-person.

5 "The Rights of Wild Rice," CELDF, February 8, 2019, https://celdf.org /2019/02/the-rights-of-wild-rice.

6 John Feldman, *Symbiotic Earth: How Lynn Margulis Rocked the Boat and Started a Scientific Revolution Online*, 2019, https://vimeo.com/ondemand/symbioticearthhv.

7 J. B. MacKinnon, *The Once and Future World: Nature as It Was, as It Is, as It Could Be* (Vintage Canada, 2014), 167–68.

8 Jose Iriarte et al., "The Origins of Amazonian Landscapes: Plant Cultivation, Domestication and the Spread of Food Production in Tropical South America," *Quaternary Science Reviews* 248 (November 2020): 106582, https://doi.org/10.1016/j.quascirev.2020.106582.

9 MacKinnon, *Once and Future World*, 181–88.

10 Francisco Sánchez-Bayo and Kris A. G. Wyckhuys, "Worldwide Decline of the Entomofauna: A Review of Its Drivers," *Biological Conservation* 232 (April 2019): 8–27, https://doi.org/10.1016/j.biocon.2019.01.020.

11 "Nearly 3 Billion Birds Gone," Cornell Lab of Ornithology, Cornell University, September 2019, www.birds.cornell.edu/home/bring-birds-back.

12 John W. Fitzpatrick and Peter P. Marra, "The Crisis for Birds Is a Crisis for Us All," *New York Times*, September 19, 2019, www.nytimes.com/2019/09/19/opinion/crisis-birds-north-america.html.

13 Scott Simon, "Opinion: 1 Million Species Are at Risk of Disappearing. Humans Should Act Now," NPR, May 11, 2019, www.npr.org/2019/05/11/722299062/opinion-one-million-species-are-at-risk-of-disappearing-humans-should-act-now.

14 Camilo Mora et al., "How Many Species Are There on Earth and in the Ocean?," *PLoS Biology* 9, no. 8 (August 23, 2011), https://doi.org/10.1371/journal.pbio.1001127.

15 Megan Sauer, "Elon Musk: 'I'll Be Surprised If We're Not Landing on Mars Within Five Years,'" CNBC, December 15, 2021, www.cnbc.com/2021/12/15/elon-musk-surprised-if-were-not-landing-on-mars-within-five-years.html.

Chapter 7. We Are Nature

1 George MacKerron and Susana Mourato, "Happiness Is Greater in Natural Environments," *Global Environmental Change* 23, no. 5 (October 2013): 992–1000, https://doi.org/10.1016/j.gloenvcha.2013.03.010.

2 Lance A. Wallace, "The Total Exposure Assessment Methodology (TEAM) Study: Summary and Analysis," US Environmental Protection Agency, EPA/600/6-87/002a, June 1987, https://nepis.epa.gov/Exe/ZyPURL.cgi?Dockey=2000UC5T.TXT.

3 Mathew P. White et al., "Spending at Least 120 Minutes a Week in Nature Is Associated with Good Health and Well-Being," *Scientific Reports* 9, no. 1 (June 13, 2019), https://doi.org/10.1038/s41598-019-44097-3.

4 Marcia P. Jimenez et al., "Associations Between Nature Exposure and Health: A Review of the Evidence," *International Journal of Environmental Research and Public Health* 18, no. 9 (April 30, 2021): 4790, https://doi.org /10.3390/ijerph18094790.

5 Roger S. Ulrich, "View Through a Window May Influence Recovery from Surgery," *Science* 224, no. 4647 (April 27, 1984): 420–21, https://doi .org/10.1126/science.6143402.

6 Jonas Schwaab et al., "The Role of Urban Trees in Reducing Land Surface Temperatures in European Cities," *Nature Communications* 12, no. 1 (November 23, 2021), https://doi.org/10.1038/s41467-021-26768-w.

7 Phillip Wolff and Douglas L. Medin, "Measuring the Evolution and Devolution of Folkbiological Knowledge," Northwestern University Department of Psychology, 1999, https://groups.psych.northwestern.edu /medin/publications/wolff%20medin%20pankratz%20devolution.pdf.

8 MacKinnnon, *Once and Future World,* 5.

9 Deqiang Ma, Briana Abrahms, and Neil Carter, "Global Expansion of Human-Wildlife Overlap in the 21st Century," *Science Advances* 10, no. 34 (August 21, 2024): 7706, https://doi.org/0.1126/sciadv.adp7706.

10 Richard Schuster, Ryan R. Germain, Joseph R. Bennett, Nicholas J. Reo, and Peter Arcese, "Vertebrate Biodiversity on Indigenous-Managed Lands in Australia, Brazil, and Canada Equals That in Protected Areas," *Environmental Science & Policy* 101 (November 2019): 1–6, https://doi.org /10.1016/j.envsci.2019.07.002.

Chapter 8. Humans Are Social Animals

1 Teresa E. Seeman, "Social Ties and Health: The Benefits of Social Integration," *Annals of Epidemiology* 6, no. 5 (September 1996): 442–51, https:// doi.org/10.1016/s1047-2797(96)00095-6.

2 Vivek Murthy, "Our Epidemic of Loneliness and Isolation: The US Surgeon General's Advisory on the Healing Effects of Social Connection and Community," US Department of Health and Human Services, Office of the Surgeon General, May 2023, www.hhs.gov/sites/default/files/surgeon -general-social-connection-advisory.pdf.

3 Robin M. Williams, *American Society: A Sociological Interpretation* (Knopf, 1970).

4 Ashlesha Datar and Nancy Nicosia, "Assessing Social Contagion in Body Mass Index, Overweight, and Obesity Using a Natural Experiment," *JAMA Pediatrics* 172, no. 3 (March 1, 2018): 239, https://doi.org/10.1001 /jamapediatrics.2017.4882.

5 Christina Gough, "Global Health and Wellness Market Value 2027," *Statista,* August 19, 2024, www.statista.com/statistics/491362/health -wellness-market-value.

6 Meryl Davies, "Five Years on from the First Minister for Loneliness," *Reengage,* May 4, 2023, https://reengage.org.uk/latest-news/five-years -on-from-the-first-minister-for-loneliness. ·

7 B. Egolf, J. Lasker, S. Wolf, and L. Potvin, "The Roseto Effect: A 50-Year Comparison of Mortality Rates," *American Journal of Public Health* 82, no. 8 (August 1992): 1089–92, https://doi.org/10.2105/ajph.82.8.1089.

8 "Life Expectancy in the U.S. Declined a Year and Half in 2020," Centers for Disease Control and Prevention, July 21, 2021, www.cdc.gov/nchs /pressroom/nchs_press_releases/2021/202107.htm.

9 Vivek Hallegere Murthy, *Together: The Healing Power of Human Connection in a Sometimes Lonely World* (Harper Wave, 2023).

10 John T. Cacioppo and Stephanie Cacioppo, "Social Relationships and Health: The Toxic Effects of Perceived Social Isolation," *Social and Personality Psychology Compass* 8, no. 2 (February 2014): 58–72, https://doi .org/10.1111/spc3.12087.

11 Amartya Sen, *Development as Freedom* (Oxford University Press, 1999).

12 I. H. Yen and G. A. Kaplan, "Neighborhood Social Environment and Risk of Death: Multilevel Evidence from the Alameda County Study," *American Journal of Epidemiology* 149, no. 10 (May 15, 1999): 898–907, https://doi.org /10.1093/oxfordjournals.aje.a009733.

13 Richard G. Wilkinson and Kate Pickett, *The Inner Level: How More Equal Societies Reduce Stress, Restore Sanity and Improve Everybody's Well-Being* (Allen Lane, 2018), 1.

14 Isabel Wilkerson, *Caste: The Origins of Our Discontents* (Random House, 2023).

15 Sarah A. O. Gray et al., "Thinking Across Generations: Unique Contributions of Maternal Early Life and Prenatal Stress to Infant Physiology," *Journal of the American Academy of Child & Adolescent Psychiatry* 56, no. 11 (November 2017): 922–29, https://doi.org/10.1016/j.jaac.2017.09.001.

16 Carl Zimmer, "The Famine Ended 70 Years Ago, but Dutch Genes Still Bear Scars," *New York Times*, January 31, 2018, www.nytimes.com /2018/01/31/science/dutch-famine-genes.html.

17 Rupa Marya and Raj Patel, *Inflamed: Deep Medicine and the Anatomy of Injustice* (Picador, 2022), 215.

18 Jacob Mugumbate, "Samkange's Theory of Ubuntu and Its Contribution to a Decolonised Social Work Pedagogy," in *The Routledge Handbook of Critical Pedagogies for Social Work*, ed. Christine Morley, Phillip Ablett, Carolyn Noble, and Stephen Cowden, 412–23 (Routledge, 2020), https:// doi.org/10.4324/9781351002042-34.

19 Clarissa Pinkola Estés, "Do Not Lose Heart, We Were Made for These Times," Daily Good, March 13, 2020, www.dailygood.org/story/1538 /do-not-lose-heart-we-were-made-for-these-times-clarissa-pinkola -estes.

20 Dwane Brown, "How One Man Convinced 200 Ku Klux Klan Members to Give Up Their Robes," *NPR,* August 20, 2017, www.npr.org/2017/08/20 /544861933/how-one-man-convinced-200-ku-klux-klan-members-to -give-up-their-robes.

Chapter 9. Embracing Death

1 Lester Haines, "Magpies Hold Funerals for Fallen Feathered Friends," *The Register,* October 21, 2009, www.theregister.com/2009/10/21/magpie _funerals.

2 Wally Brown, "Traditional Navajo View on Death and Grieving," October 8, 2018, www.youtube.com/watch?v=1muGlca1ibI.

3 Eric Weiner, "Bhutan's Dark Secret to Happiness," *BBC News,* February 25, 2022, www.bbc.com/travel/article/20150408-bhutans-dark-secret -to-happiness.

4 Laura L. Carstensen, "Socioemotional Selectivity Theory: The Role of Perceived Endings in Human Motivation," *Gerontologist* 61, no. 8 (October 27, 2021): 1188–96, https://doi.org/10.1093/geront/gnab116.

5 Joan Didion, *The Year of Magical Thinking* (Alfred A Knopf, 2005).

6 Phoebe Weston, "No Birdsong, No Water in the Creek, No Beating Wings: How a Haven for Nature Fell Silent," *Guardian*, April 16, 2024, www.theguardian.com/environment/2024/apr/16/nature-silent-bernie -krause-recording-sound-californian-state-park-aoe.

7 Olivia Rosane, "Thousands of Migrating Birds Found Dead or Injured in Greece," *EcoWatch,* April 10, 2020, www.ecowatch.com/migrating -birds-dead-greece-2645686203.html.

8 Samuel B. Fey et al., "Recent Shifts in the Occurrence, Cause, and Magnitude of Animal Mass Mortality Events," *Proceedings of the National Academy of Sciences* 112, no. 4 (January 12, 2015): 1083–88, https://doi.org /10.1073/pnas.1414894112.

9 Jemimah Steinfeld, "China's Deadly Science Lesson: How an Ill-Conceived Campaign Against Sparrows Contributed to One of the Worst Famines in History," *Index on Censorship* 47, no. 3 (September 2018): 49–49, https://doi.org/10.1177/0306422018800259.

10 Marco Lambertini, *Living Planet Report 2020: Bending the Curve of Biodiversity Loss* (World Wildlife Fund Canada, 2020).

Chapter 10. Finding Hope

1 Michel Poulain et al., "Identification of a Geographic Area Characterized by Extreme Longevity in the Sardinia Island: The Akea Study," *Experimental Gerontology* 39, no. 9 (September 2004): 1423–29, https://doi .org/10.1016/j.exger.2004.06.016.

2 Anthony J. Papalas, *Rebels and Radicals: Icaria 1600–2000* (Bolchazy-Carducci, 2005), 162.

3 Norimitsu Onishi, "Urasoe Journal; on U.S. Fast Food, More Okinawans Grow Super-Sized," *New York Times*, March 30, 2004, www.nytimes.com /2004/03/30/world/urasoe-journal-on-us-fast-food-more-okinawans-grow -super-sized.html.

4 Michel Poulain, "Exceptional Longevity in Okinawa," *Demographic Research* 25 (July 21, 2011): 245–84, https://doi.org/10.4054/demres.2011.25.7.

5 Marya and Patel, *Inflamed*, 141–44.

Chapter 11. The Path Forward

1 Suzanne Simard, *Finding the Mother Tree: Discovering the Wisdom of the Forest* (Vintage Books, 2021).

2 Ruby Prosser Scully, "Tree Stumps That Should Be Dead Can Be Kept Alive by Nearby Trees," *New Scientist*, July 25, 2019, www.newscientist. com/article/2211209-tree-stumps-that-should-be-dead-can-be-kept-alive -by-nearby-trees.

3 Thomas D. Seeley, *Honeybee Democracy* (Princeton University Press, 2010), 73–98.

4 Seeley, *Honeybee Democracy*, 75–76.

5 Richard Gerrig and Mahzarin Banaji, "Language and Thought," in *Thinking and Problem Solving*, ed. Robert J. Sternberg, 233–61 (Academic Press, 1994).

6 Wade Davis, *The Wayfinders: Why Ancient Wisdom Matters in the Modern World* (House of Anansi, 2009), 3.

7 *Merriam-Webster Collegiate*, s.v. "wilderness," www.merriam-webster.com /dictionary/wilderness.

8 *The Oxford Dictionary of Phrase and Fable*, 2nd ed., s.v. "nature," www .oxfordreference.com/display/10.1093/acref/9780198609810.001.0001 /acref-9780198609810-e-4825.

9 Jeff Grignon and Robin Wall Kimmerer, "Listening to the Forest," in *Wildness: Relations of People and Place,* ed. Gavin Van Horn and John Hausdoerffer (University of Chicago Press, 2017), 65–74.

10 Lyanda Lynn Haupt, *Rooted: Life at the Crossroads of Science, Nature, and Spirit* (Little, Brown Spark, 2021), 26.

11 Enrique Salmon, "Kincentric Ecology: Indigenous Perceptions of the Human-Nature Relationship," *Ecological Applications* 10, no. 5 (October 2000): 1327, https://doi.org/10.2307/2641288.

12 John Hausdoerffer, "The *Akiing* Ethic: Seeking Ancestral Wildness Beyond Aldo Leopold's Wilderness," in *Wildness: Relations of People and Place,* ed. Gavin Van Horn and John Hausdoerffer (University of Chicago Press, 2017), 195–204.

13 Joy Donnell, "Creating Harmonious Lives—Hozho and Lyla June John-ston," May 16, 2020, http://doitinpublic.com/creating-harmonious-lives -hozho-and-lyla-june-johnston.

14 J. N. B. Hewitt, "Orenda and a Definition of Religion," *American Anthro-pologist* 4, no. 1 (January–March 1902): 33–46, https://doi.org/10.1525 /aa.1902.4.1.02a00050.

15 Robin Wall Kimmerer, "Speaking of Nature," *Orion*, 2017, https:// orionmagazine.org/article/speaking-of-nature.

16 Geert Hofstede, "Dimensionalizing Cultures: The Hofstede Model in Con-text," *Online Readings in Psychology and Culture* 2, no. 1 (December 1, 2011), https://doi.org/10.9707/2307-0919.1014.

17 Daniel J. Siegel, *Intraconnected: Mwe (Me + We) as the Integration of Self, Identity, and Belonging* (W. W. Norton, 2023).

18 Alison Jane Martingano, "Social Media and Empathy Around the Globe," *Psychology Today*, May 9, 2023, www.psychologytoday.com/us/blog/what -do-you-mean/202305/social-media-and-empathy-around-the-globe.

19 Kimmerer, "Speaking of Nature."

20 Kimmerer, *Braiding Sweetgrass*, 214.

21 Enrique Salmon, "Teaching Kincentric Ecology in an Urban Environment," *Journal of Sustainability Education*, November 2015, www.susted.com /wordpress/content/teaching-kincentric-ecology-in-an-urban-environment _2015_11.

22 Hausdoerffer, "*Akiing* Ethic," 195–204.

Chapter 12. Possible Futures

1 Hannah Comtesse et al., "Ecological Grief as a Response to Environmen-tal Change: A Mental Health Risk or Functional Response?," *International Journal of Environmental Research and Public Health* 18, no. 2 (January 16, 2021): 734, https://doi.org/10.3390/ijerph18020734.

2 Alan Neuhauser, "100,000 Americans Die from Air Pollution, Study Finds," *US News & World Report*, April 8, 2019, www.usnews.com/news/national -news/articles/2019-04-08/100-000-americans-die-from-air-pollution -study-finds.

3 Sandro Galea et al., "Estimated Deaths Attributable to Social Factors in the United States," *American Journal of Public Health* 101, no. 8 (August 2011): 1456–65, https://doi.org/10.2105/ajph.2010.300086.

4 John Vidal, "Environmental Risks Killing 12.6 Million People, WHO Study Says," *Guardian*, March 15, 2016, www.theguardian.com/environment/2016 /mar/15/environmental-risks-killing-126-million-people-who-study-says.

5 Christiana Figueres and Tom Rivett-Carnac, *The Future We Choose: Surviving the Climate Crisis* (Alfred A. Knopf, 2020), 7.

6 adrienne maree brown, *Emergent Strategy: Shaping Change, Changing Worlds* (AK Press, 2017), 19.
7 Kim Stanley Robinson, *The Ministry for the Future* (Orbit, 2022).
8 Octavia E. Butler, *Parable of the Sower* (Warner Books, 1999).
9 Charlotte McConaghy, *Migrations* (Flatiron Books, 2020).
10 Eric Holthaus, *The Future Earth: A Radical Vision for What's Possible in the Age of Warming* (HarperOne, 2020), 103.
11 Ursula K. Le Guin, *Always Coming Home* (HarperCollins, 1985).
12   *Merriam-Webster Collegiate*, s.v. "ark," www.merriam-webster.com /dictionary/ark.
13 William deBuys, *The Trail to Kanjiroba: Rediscovering Earth in an Age of Loss* (Seven Stories Press, 2021), 175.

Chapter 13. Acting Collectively

1 Charles Clements, *Witness to War: An American Doctor in El Salvador* (Bantam Books, 1984).
2 John Schmal, "Chiapas: Forever Indigenous," Indigenous Mexico, May 12, 2024, www.indigenousmexico.org/articles/chiapas-forever-indigenous.
3 Hilary Klein, "A Spark of Hope: The Ongoing Lessons of the Zapatista Revolution 25 Years On," *NACLA,* January 18, 2019, https://nacla.org /news/2022/12/21/spark-hope-ongoing-lessons-zapatista-revolution-25-years.
4 "El Despertador Mexicano" (Zapatista Manifesto), Rethinking History and the Nation State: Mexico and the United States, December 31, 1993, http://archive.oah.org/special-issues/mexico/zapmanifest.html.
5 Klein, "A Spark of Hope."
6 John Vidal, "Mexico's Zapatista Rebels, 24 Years on and Defiant in Mountain Strongholds," *Guardian*, February 17, 2018, www.theguardian.com/global -development/2018/feb/17/mexico-zapatistas-rebels-24-years-mountain -strongholds.
7 "2015: Seguir Con Lo Mismo o Avanzar a Otros Mundos Posibles.- Entrevista Con Omar García, De Ayotzinapa," Radio Zapatista, December 31, 2014, https://radiozapatista.org/?p=11573.
8 adrienne maree brown, *Emergent Strategy: Shaping Change, Changing Worlds* (AK Press, 2017), 18.
9 Nick Estes, *Our History Is the Future: Standing Rock Versus the Dakota Access Pipeline, and the Long Tradition of Indigenous Resistance* (Verso, 2019), 252.
10 "Yale Climate Opinion Maps 2023," Yale Program on Climate Change Communication, August 21, 2024, https://climatecommunication.yale.edu /visualizations-data/ycom-us.
11 "Fracking Bans and Moratoriums," Local Progress, n.d., accessed September 4, 2024, https://localprogress.org/wp-content/uploads/2013/09

/Fracking-Bans-and-Moratoriums.pdf; Héctor Herrera, "The Legal Status of Fracking Worldwide: An Environmental Law and Human Rights Perspective," GNHRE, n.d., accessed September 3, 2024, https://gnhre .org/?p=10555.

12 brown, *Emergent Strategy*, 13.

13 Eric S. Kim et al., "Sense of Purpose in Life and Five Health Behaviors in Older Adults," *Preventive Medicine* 139 (October 2020): 106172, https://doi .org/10.1016/j.ypmed.2020.106172.

Epilogue: The Coyote and the Cottonwood

1 Daniel Kahneman and Angus Deaton, "High Income Improves Evaluation of Life but Not Emotional Well-Being," *Proceedings of the National Academy of Sciences* 107, no. 38 (September 7, 2010): 16489–93, https:// doi.org/10.1073/pnas.1011492107.

2 Lynsey A. White and Stanley D. Gehrt, "Coyote Attacks on Humans in the United States and Canada," *Human Dimensions of Wildlife* 14, no. 6 (November 30, 2009): 419–32, https://doi.org/10.1080/10871200903055326.

3 Sarah Hojsak, "Finding Beauty in a Broken World with Terry Tempest Williams," Drexel University, April 14, 2023, https://drexel.edu/coas/news -events/news/2023/April/terry-tempest-williams-recap.

4 Estes, "Do Not Lose Heart."

Index

About the Author

Dr. Wendy Johnson, MD, MPH, is a clinician, public health expert, activist, and writer whose career includes stints scaling up HIV treatment in Mozambique, overseeing an urban public health department in Cleveland, Ohio, and directing a community clinic in Santa Fe, New Mexico. She currently practices family and addiction medicine, serving patients in rural northern New Mexico for El Centro Family Health, and also consults with community clinics in Appalachian Ohio. As an assistant professor in both the University of Washington's Global Health Department and the University of New Mexico Medical School's Department of Family and Community Medicine, she teaches and mentors medical and public health students and residents. Dr. Johnson grew up along the shores of Lake Erie in Buffalo, Cleveland, and Toledo and currently resides outside of Santa Fe in a community that includes two dogs, many human neighbors, a few bears, and countless coyotes and cottonwoods.

About North Atlantic Books

North Atlantic Books (NAB) is an independent, nonprofit publisher committed to a bold exploration of the relationships between mind, body, spirit, and nature. Founded in 1974, NAB aims to nurture a holistic view of the arts, sciences, humanities, and healing. To make a donation or to learn more about our books, authors, events, and newsletter, please visit www .northatlanticbooks.com.